Breastfeeding Special Care Babies

Breastfeeding Special Care Babies

Sandra Lang

MPhil, RM, RGN, Dip. Ed, Cert Ed, ENB 405
Senior Lecturer, Department of Midwifery Studies,
University of Central Lancashire

 The Neonatal Nurses' Association

Baillière Tindall
London · Philadelphia · Toronto
Sydney · Tokyo

BAILLIÈRE TINDALL W.B. SAUNDERS
24–28 Oval Road
London NW1 7DX

The Curtis Center
Independence Square West
Philadelphia, PA 19106–3399, USA

Harcourt Brace & Company
56 Horner Avenue
Toronto, Ontario M8Z 4X6, Canada

Harcourt Brace & Company, Australia
30–52 Smidmore Street,
Marrickville, NSW 2204, Australia

Harcourt Brace & Company, Japan
Ichibancho Central Building
22–1 Ichibancho
Chiyoda-ku, Tokyo 101, Japan

A catalogue record for this book is available from the British Library

ISBN 0–7020–2020–6

Typeset by Wyvern Typesetting Ltd, Bristol
Printed in Great Britain by WBC Book Manufacturers,
Bridgend, Mid Glamorgan

Contents

Forewords   xiii
Acknowledgements   xvii
Katy – A Special Baby   xix
Introduction   xxi

Chapter 1 – The basics of breastfeeding
1.1 The challenge of breastfeeding   1
1.2 The benefits of breastfeeding   2
    1.2.1 Benefits to the baby   3
    1.2.2 Benefits to the mother   3
    1.2.3 The benefits of the breastmilk   4
1.3 Anatomy and physiology of the lactating breast   4
    1.3.1 The initiation of lactation   5
    1.3.2 Artificial stimulation of lactation   6
1.4 The composition and sequence of milk production   7
    1.4.1 Appearance of the stages of milk
           production   7
    1.4.2 The composition of breastmilk   7
           Colostrum   8
           Mature human milk   9
1.5 The development of a baby's feeding ability   13
1.6 Factors affecting a baby's ability to feed efficiently   15
References   17

**Chapter 2 – The position and attachment of the baby
           at the breast**
2.1 Positioning and breast attachment   21
    2.1.1 Positioning, monitoring and oxygen
           therapy   21
    2.1.2 Before positioning and attaching the baby
           at the breast   22
    2.1.3 Positions for breastfeeding   25

The 'underarm' position   26
The 'traditional' position   28
Other useful positions   29
Breastfeeding more than one baby at each
feed   30
2.1.4   Breast attachment   30
2.1.5   How to remove a baby from the breast   32
2.1.6   How to help a baby with difficulty
        attaching to the breast   33
2.1.7   How to attach a baby to the breast who
        has become used to a bottle teat or dummy 34
2.2   How long should a feed last?   34
2.2.1   Remedies to use when feeding times are
        prolonged   35
2.3   How often should a baby feed?   37
2.3.1   The preterm baby   38
2.4   Has the baby had sufficient?   38
2.5   The baby's need for oral stimulation   39
References   42

Chapter 3 – The expression of breastmilk
3.1   Hand expression   43
3.1.1   When and how often to hand express   44
3.1.2   How to hand express   45
        The principles of hand expression   46
        Possible additions to and variations of the
        principles of hand expression   48
        What to expect at an individual expression
        session   49
3.1.3   How to teach a mother to hand express   50
        Practical instruction   51
3.2   When and how to use a mechanical pump   52
3.2.1   When to pump   52
        How often?   53
        How long?   53
        The amount of milk produced   53
3.2.2   How to pump   54
3.3   Storage of expressed breastmilk and its sequence
      of use   56
3.3.1   Containers and storage   56
        The effect of the container on milk
        composition   57
3.3.2   Defrosting breastmilk   57

3.3.3 Sequence of breastmilk use 58
3.4 Prolonged expression of breastmilk 58
 3.4.1 Suggestions for reducing long-term
  problems 59
  Back massage 60
 3.4.2 How to stop using a pump 63
  Weaning off the pump 63
3.5 Types of pump 65
3.6 Breast massage 65
 3.6.1 Why is it necessary? 65
 3.6.2 How to massage 66
  Method 1 66
  Method 2 67
  Other methods of massage 67
3.7 Supplementary and replacement (complementary)
 feeding 69
 3.7.1 When supplementary or replacement feeds
  are necessary 70
3.8 Breast shells/drip catchers 71
References 72

Chapter 4 – Breast conditions
4.1 How to cope with engorgement 74
 4.1.1 Initial fullness of the breast 74
 4.1.2 Milk engorgement 75
4.2 Cracked and sore nipples 76
 4.2.1 Sore nipples (pink/red with no cracks) 76
  At the time of feeding 77
  Between feeds or expressing 77
 4.2.2 Nipples that are cracked and sore 78
4.3 Inverted and flat nipples 79
 4.3.1 Management of inverted or flat nipples 80
4.4 Blocked ducts, lobes, mastitis and breast abscess 82
 4.4.1 Blocked ducts and lobes 82
  Signs of blocked ducts and lobes 82
  Treatment 83
  Prevention 84
 4.4.2 Mastitis 84
  Signs of mastitis 84
  Treatment 85
 4.4.3 Breast abscess 85
  Signs of breast abscess 85

Treatment   86
4.5   Breastfeeding and nipple shields   86
       4.5.1   How to avoid the use of nipple shields   86
       4.5.2   Situations in which a nipple shield may be
               appropriate   88
       4.5.3   How to use nipple shields   89
       4.5.4   How to wean a baby off the shield   89
References   90

Chapter 5 – The milk supply
5.1   Too little milk   92
       5.1.1   Physical factors that may interfere with, or
               cause low milk production   93
       5.1.2   Suggested remedies   93
5.2   Too much milk and leaking breasts   96
       5.2.1   Leaking breasts   97
5.3   Expression of the fat-rich hind-milk   99
       5.3.1   Promotion of weight gain and growth in
               preterm babies   100
       5.3.2   The formula   100
               Example   100
               Important points to remember when
               expressing   101
       5.3.3   Promotion of weight gain in breastfeeding
               babies   102
5.4   The normal growth of the breastfed baby   102
5.5   Weight loss and test weighing   103
       5.5.1   Causes of weight loss   103
       5.5.2   Test weighing   103
5.6   Breast surgery and feeding   104
5.7   Relactation   105
       5.7.1   Relactation if the mother has produced
               breastmilk previously   106
       5.7.2   Relactation if the mother has never
               produced breastmilk previously   107
5.8   The mother's diet and fluids   107
References   108

Chapter 6 – Breastfeeding the vulnerable baby
6.1   Tongue tie   111
6.2   Cleft lip and/or palate   111
       6.2.1   Cleft lip   112
       6.2.2   Cleft palate   112

6.2.3 Cleft lip and palate 114
6.2.4 The establishment of breastfeeding 114
6.2.5 If breastfeeding is not established 116
6.2.6 Support groups 116
6.2.7 General advice 117
6.3 Bell's palsy and breastfeeding 118
6.4 Breastfeeding the baby compromised by
respiratory and heart problems 119
6.5 Multiple births 121
6.6 The preterm baby 121
6.6.1 Overcoming the problems 122
6.7 The ventilated baby 124
6.8 The jaundiced baby 125
6.8.1 Physiological or idiopathic jaundice 125
6.8.2 How to reduce the development of
jaundice in the first few days after birth 125
6.8.3 Pathological or haemolytic jaundice 126
6.8.4 Phototherapy and feeding method 126
6.8.5 Breastmilk jaundice 127
6.9 The unsettled baby 127
6.10 Hypoglycaemia and the breastfed baby 129
6.10.1 Which babies are at risk? 129
High-risk factors 130
Low-risk factors 130
6.10.2 Breastfeeding and the low-risk baby 130
6.10.3 Breastfeeding and the high-risk baby 131
6.11 Bowels and the breastfed baby 132
6.11.1 Colour and consistency 132
6.11.2 Warning signs 132
6.11.3 Frequency of bowel actions 133
6.12 Thrush and breastfeeding 133
6.13 HIV and breastfeeding 133
References 134

Chapter 7 – Alternative methods of feeding and
breastfeeding
7.1 Alternative and supplementary methods of
feeding 136
7.2 Gastric and transpyloric tubes 136
7.2.1 Transpyloric tubes 136
7.2.2 Gastric tubes 137
7.2.3 Continuous and 1–2 hourly bolus
tube-feeding 137

Continuous pump feeds 137
1–2 hourly bolus tube-feeding 138
7.2.4 Breastfeeding and gastric tubes 139
Continuous gastric tube feeds 140
1–2 hourly bolus gastric tube feeds 140
3 hourly bolus gastric tube feeds 141
When formula milk has to be used 141
7.3 Direct expression of breastmilk 141
7.4 Cup-feeding 143
7.4.1 General reasons for using a cup 143
Advantages of cup-feeding 144
Disadvantages of cup-feeding 144
7.4.2 When and how to use a cup 144
The preterm baby 145
The term baby 146
7.4.3 The baby with special requirements 147
The baby with a cleft lip and/or cleft
palate 147
The baby who cannot suck effectively 147
7.4.4 How much should the baby take? 148
7.4.5 Method of cup-feeding 149
What to use in hospital 149
What to use at home 149
Method for feeding 149
Type of milk to use 150
7.5 The nursing supplementer 150
7.5.1 Method 152
7.5.2 How to make a nursing supplementer 153
7.5.3 Long-term use of the nursing supplementer 154
7.6 Syringes and droppers 154
7.7 Finger 'assessment' of feeding 155
7.7.1 Method 156
7.8 The bottle 156
7.8.1 Preterm babies and bottle-feeding 158
7.8.2 Bottle teats, dummies and the vulnerable
baby 158
7.9 Mixed breast- and bottle-feeding 158
References 159

Chapter 8 – Breastfeeding and common drugs
8.1 Breastfeeding and drugs 161
8.1.1 Some common drugs to avoid 162
The combined contraceptive pill 162

	Caffeine	162
	Nicotine	163
8.2	Breastfeeding and maternal medication	163
8.2.1	Medication with contraindications to breastfeeding	163
8.2.2	Medication with which breastfeeding can be continued	163
References		164

Chapter 9 – Recommendations for the support of breastfeeding
9.1 Recommendations for the support of breastfeeding on a neonatal or specialist paediatric unit   166
  9.1.1 Staff education   166
  9.1.2 The neonatal unit   168
  9.1.3 Helping the parents   169
References   170

Appendix – Breastfeeding support
  Breastfeeding support groups   171
  Other useful addresses   171
  Useful literature   171
    Books   171
    Other literature   172

Index   173

This book is dedicated to Katy and Marcus,
two very special babies,
to the many other 'special' babies and their families,
and the nursing and medical staff, past and present,
of the Exeter Neonatal Unit

Foreword

Breastfeeding Special Care Babies fills a gap in the literature of breastfeeding. It provides a comprehensive guide for staff in neonatal units and midwives.

The book fulfils the promise made in the Introduction, offering a range of conventional and unconventional approaches to feeding the preterm, sick and other vulnerable babies.

Included in the first two chapters are the essential factors which govern a baby's ability to feed and his ability to do so effectively. This leads into the practical aspects of breastfeeding, described clearly and with specific application to the preterm baby.

An excellent chapter on expressing breastmilk follows, detailing hand expression, storage and effect of storage and freezing breastmilk. To reduce problems for mothers who express milk over a long period of time, the author describes back-massage to stimulate the release of oxytocin and the 'let-down' reflex.

Common breastfeeding problems are dealt with succinctly and include the disadvantages of the all too common use of nipple shields in Chapter 4, and Chapter 5 includes helpful descriptions of relactation. In Chapter 6 milk production is described, and is related to milk expression and the nutritional needs for growth of the low birth weight and sick baby.

For babies with particular feeding problems, for example, babies with cleft palate, Bell's palsy, respiratory and heart problems, alternative methods of feeding are given in great detail with advice on how any difficulties can often be overcome. Midwives will find the sections on physiological jaundice and the use of phototherapy particularly useful, as well as the helpful suggestions on the unsettled baby. An outline of the effect of drugs on breastfeeding refers also to other documents to be consulted for their effects.

Concluding the book are excellent recommendations for the management of breastfeeding on a neonatal or specialist paediatric unit.

Many aspects of breastfeeding wait to be researched, including some of the techniques and skills mentioned. However, common sense always prevails. Tender, loving care and respect of the mother and baby shines through all sections.

I would recommend this book without hesitation.

Dora Henschel, RN, RM, MTD, IBCLC
Co-ordinator of the Joint Breastfeeding Initiative

Foreword

The old adage 'Breast is Best' is a well used phrase. However, if breastfeeding a well term baby is complex then it is doubly so if the baby is sick or pre-term.

The reasons why women give up breastfeeding have been studied extensively and it is now axiomatic to state that lack of support coupled with conflicting advice often heralds failure. Appropriate and sensitive advice can be pivotal in encouraging mothers to feed their babies.

Health professionals need updating with research related to breastfeeding and, when possible, to have clear rationales for the actions we recommend. We must be willing to explore new techniques and initiatives – a sound knowledge base will increase the confidence of the practitioner and in turn enable the mother to feel more confident in her own skill.

As neonatal nurses and midwives we have a daunting responsibility, for the care and advice which we provide has such a powerful impact on the mother–child relationship. Breastfeeding is a major part of that relationship and this book will join the Royal College of Midwives publication *Successful Breastfeeding* and the WHO/UNICEF *Ten Steps to Successful Breastfeeding* in providing clear guidelines to promote success.

For many reasons it may not be possible or appropriate for the babies in our care to be breastfed. However, when it is possible the art and science of breastfeeding are not easy to teach or learn. Sandra Lang's book will be useful to those responsible for education as well as practitioners. The Neonatal Nurses' Association welcome it as a resource for both neonatal nurses and midwives alike as part of an armoury of information for the families we care for.

Jackie Dent, BSc, RGN, RM, RCNT, JBCNS 400, ADM, Cert Ed
Chairperson, Neonatal Nurses' Association Education Group

Acknowledgements

I would like to thank the following people who have shared with me their professional expertise, wisdom and enthusiasm for breastfeeding – they have contributed a great deal to this book: Nola Gendle, Mary-Anne Shields, Marlene Harris, Pamela Bell, Tracy Caan, Sharon Hore, Dr Marie Hanlon, Helen Shoesmith and all the Midwifery, Nursing and Medical Staff at the Exeter Neonatal Unit; the Breastfeeding Counsellors from the Exeter Branch of the National Childbirth Trust; Dora Henschel; The Royal College of Midwives Breastfeeding Working Group, particularly Chloe Fisher and Sally Inch for their helpful suggestions and advice; and the Neonatal Nurses Association.

I owe special thanks to Gabriella Palmer for her wonderful way with words and her generosity in helping me to express clearly some of the more complex parts of the text.

I am also grateful to Fiona Dykes and Kate Dinwoodie of the Department of Midwifery Studies at the University of Central Lancashire; Liz Jones of the North Staffs Neonatal unit and Harold Hirsch of Egnell-Ameda for the photographs used in this book; and to Daphne Paley-Smith for her lovely line drawings.

My thanks also go to my friends and family for their support and encouragement, and to my colleagues in the Department of Midwifery Studies at the University of Central Lancashire – who probably know this book by heart!

I have left two very special acknowledgements until last. Early in the 1970s, I travelled to a town called Janakpur in southern Nepal as a volunteer with the Volunteer Service Overseas. It was here and in the surrounding villages that I spent many hours behind mud walls with the women and children in their compounds. I observed and learned about the subtle art of breastfeeding, and saw the alternative methods that were used to feed babies born either prematurely or very small, and who were unable to breastfeed exclusively at birth. Many of these babies survived because of the skill of their mothers in using cups and rudimentary nursing supplementers. All of them eventually succeeded in breastfeeding. I do not know or remember the names of many of these women or their babies who taught me so much, but I am deeply grateful for the education I received from them.

Finally, I am indebted to the many mothers, fathers and babies whose experiences of breastfeeding have made this book possible.

Sandra Lang

Katy – A Special Baby

The baby on the front cover is Katy Taylor. She and her parents have contributed more to this book than they will ever realise, and I am grateful to her parents for giving permission to use her photograph.

Katy was born at 24 weeks gestation on the 23 March 1990, weighing 756 grammes. She was ventilated for a total of 48 days from birth and required oxygen via a headbox for a further 15 days, before having oxygen via nasal cannulae. This was eventually discontinued **one month** after discharge. She was in the Neonatal Intensive Care Unit for a total of 74 days, before being transferred to the Special Care Unit for low dependency care.

She was initially fed intravenously. She began to have expressed breastmilk on day 4 via a nasal gastric tube at 1/2 ml per hour. Thereafter she received:

- Continuous pump feeds for 51 days from day 4 to day 54
- 1-hourly bolus feeds for 9 days from day 55 to day 63
- 2-hourly bolus feeds for 8 days from day 64 to day 71
- 3-hourly bolus feeds for 11 days from day 72 to day 82
- 3–4-hourly bolus feeds (as required) for 27 days from day 83 to day 104 and was breastfeeding on demand from day 105

Her breastfeeding history

- On day 48 she had her first 'lick' at the breast (this was also the day on which she was extubated). She was approximately 31 weeks old.
- On day 49 she had a few gentle sucks at the breast.
- On day 52 she had a short breastfeed (requiring supplementing by gastric tube).

- On day 59 she had 2 slightly longer breastfeeds (requiring supplementing by gastric tube).
- Between days 60 to 102 she was having at least 1–4 breastfeeds a day. The nasal tube was gradually removed with occasional oral tube feeds given.
- On day 74 she had her first cup-feed. Altogether, she had 38 cup-feeds during the next 29 days. Amounts taken were between 5 and 85 ml. The majority of the cup-feeds were in excess of her fluid requirement as charted.
- On day 103 she no longer required any tube- or cup-feeds, for she was then totally breastfed.
- By day 105 she was demand feeding approximately every $2\frac{1}{2}$–4 hours.
- She was discharged weighing 2532 grammes, on day 115.

Katy is now at school, and she is considered to be very bright. She goes horse-riding, cycling and loves her ballet class. She is tall for her age and has been remarkably healthy, having to be hospitalized only once since she was discharged from the neonatal unit.

Katy stopped breastfeeding completely when she was three and a half years old.

Introduction

This is a book about breastfeeding in adversity! It is a practical guide, which has grown out of the many and varied experiences of:

- Mothers and fathers, whose babies were admitted to a neonatal unit;
- The health professionals, who with patience, imagination and skill helped many of the babies to begin life nourished with their mother's own breastmilk, and go home successfully breastfeeding; and
- Lay breastfeeding counsellors and health professionals, who provided continuing support to the families for a long time after the babies had gone home.

Many of the practices considered in the following chapters are fundamental to successful breastfeeding, for example, correct positioning and attachment. Many are supported by good scientific evidence, but there remain some practices, which have grown out of practical experience in a neonatal or paediatric unit, where breastfeeding may not be straightforward. Some of these practices have proven beneficial in helping both the mother and baby to establish breastfeeding – they are, therefore, also included in this book. These practices include using the nursing supplementer, the cup, and back massage. As a result, this book offers a range of conventional and unconventional approaches to the many challenging situations which can arise in hospital units caring for preterm, sick and other vulnerable babies. It is aimed at protecting the unique role of the mother who, having made the commitment to breastfeed, has a right to succeed!

1 The basics of breastfeeding

1.1 The challenge of breastfeeding

There is little doubt that breastfeeding is by far the best way to feed a term, healthy baby. Few people would also doubt that breastmilk is very important to the needs of the preterm and sick baby. Indeed, the case for the most fragile babies in our neonatal and paediatric units receiving breastmilk is persuasively made in a number of scientific articles.[1] After all, when it is considered that breastmilk contains factors which protect babies against infection, factors which aid their growth and neurological development, factors which make them less susceptible to certain diseases in childhood and even into adulthood – and incidentally has health benefits for their mothers as well, it seems illogical not to use it as a very vital part of the babies' medication and treatment.

It could be argued that breastmilk is equally as important to the long-term well-being of a vulnerable baby, as the ventilation is to the baby's short-term survival. Clear guidance on how the breastmilk is obtained and how it is fed to a baby are, therefore, essential if its benefits are to be realized.

To have a baby admitted to a neonatal or paediatric unit, for whatever reason, is a stressful and frequently frightening experience for parents. They are often confused by the technology and environment, they may feel guilty, afraid for the future and for their baby's survival or long-term outcome. Moreover, it is not unusual for the mother herself to be unwell as a result of complications during pregnancy or labour. All of which can lead to the mother feeling very insecure and to her losing confidence in her ability to care for her baby.

Therefore, when a mother has made a commitment to breastfeed, it is essential that she can be fully supported by knowledgeable and skilled health professionals who appreciate her unique role in providing not only a source of nourishment for her baby, but a very important component of the baby's treatment as well. The mother is often as vulnerable emotionally in a neonatal or paediatric unit as her baby is clinically: she needs the reassurance that her contribution is very special indeed when her baby is unable, for whatever reason, to breastfeed from the time of birth. For it is only the mother who is able to:

- Provide a 'tailor-made' food, with its own specific antibodies and other protective properties.
- Soothe her baby by holding him next to her breast, nourish him and, at the same time, provide comfort.
- Begin, through breastfeeding, to build up a close and loving relationship.

No health professional can ever provide these important human needs. Therefore, a partnership in which parents and health professionals value the role of the other in equal measure is essential to the short- and long-term well-being of the mother and her baby.

Many mothers do not succeed in breastfeeding in a neonatal unit. Some cite the lack of support from medical and nursing staff as part of the reason, some cite the conflicting advice they are given and some the lack of practical help they receive. To be quite certain that we can help mothers to succeed in breastfeeding, the information contained in the rest of this chapter and in the following chapters is aimed at overcoming the obstacles which may occur during a baby's stay in a neonatal or paediatric unit and when the baby goes home.

1.2 The benefits of breastfeeding

Breastmilk is so much more than simply nutrition, it is a unique and very complex fluid containing well over 100 documented constituents. Many scientific papers examining its biochemical properties have been written and new discoveries about its properties are constantly being made. It is considered to be a 'living fluid',[2] for in addition to its nutrient content it contains anti-bacterial, anti-viral, anti-infective and anti-parasitic factors, as well as hormones, enzymes, specialized growth factors and immunological properties.[3]

The benefits of breastfeeding are many. On a global level it significantly reduces infant morbidity and mortality,[4] and probably contributes far more to the health and well-being of a nation than perhaps is realized or acknowledged.

1.2.1 Benefits to the baby

Breastmilk and breastfeeding provides a baby with a number of important short- and long-term benefits. These include:

- A reduced incidence of gastrointestinal and respiratory infections during the neonatal period.[5,6]
- Increased protection against dental caries, and possibly less malocclusion.[7]
- A lower incidence of otitis media.[8,9]
- A lower incidence of juvenile onset diabetes.[10,11]
- Recent research indicates that breastmilk given to a preterm baby may contain factors important in the development of the brain, and central nervous system.[12,13]
- A reduced mortality rate among preterm and low birthweight babies from necrotizing enterocolitis.[14]
- It is suggested that the incidence of some childhood cancers is reduced (lymphoma and Hodgkin's disease).[15]
- Certain allergic conditions may be less severe.[16]

1.2.2 Benefits to the mother

There is increasing evidence of long-term health benefits from breastfeeding for the mother also. These include:

- A reduction in the incidence of premenopausal breast cancer and some forms of ovarian cancer.[17-19]
- A lower incidence of hip fractures in women over the age of 65.[20]
- A delay in the return of fertility.[21, 22]
- Helping the mother to lose weight naturally.[23]

In the first few days after birth the increased release of the hormones, prolactin and oxytocin, helps the uterus to return to its normal size more quickly, thus reducing the risk of serious haemorrhage in the post-natal period. Some mothers may experience the process of uterine involution as lower abdominal pain (after-pains) and/or increased loss of blood during feeding or milk expression. These events are both normal (with 'after-pains' being more common in mothers breastfeeding after a second pregnancy than after a first pregnancy).

The psychological benefits to the relationship between the mother and her baby are of paramount importance. Breastfeeding is not simply a form of nutrition, but is part of the 'nurturing' process, fundamental to the overall well-being of the family group – and as such has benefits for all of society.

1.2.3   The benefits of the breastmilk

- Breast milk is cheap and there is no waste.
- It is always at the correct temperature.
- It is ready when needed and requires no preparation.
- It is portable.
- It is easy to give at night.
- For a term baby, the milk is nutritionally perfect.

1.3   Anatomy and physiology of the lactating breast

The breasts are remarkable glands. They are capable of producing sufficient milk to sustain a baby's nutritional needs totally for the first 4–6 months of life,[24] and are capable of making a valuable contribution to the baby's diet for several more months or even years.

The breasts are composed of 15–25 lobes of glandular tissue, with each lobe containing thousands of alveoli, which are clusters of tiny 'sacs' in which the milk is stored after being produced by the glandular epithelial cells of the breast. The hormone **prolactin** makes these cells produce milk. The 'sacs' are surrounded by muscle cells (myoepithelial cells) arranged in a 'basket'-like weave. It is the hormone **oxytocin** that makes these muscles contract and squeezes the milk out into ducts which lead from the alveoli into the 10–15 distendable ducts, the **lactiferous sinuses**. When babies suckle, they compress these sinuses between their tongues and hard palates, by means of a 'wave'-like movement of their tongues. The milk is forced into the narrow ducts, which lead out on to the surface of the nipple and is then ejected (see Fig. 1.1).

Not all the lobes of the breast are productive during the com-

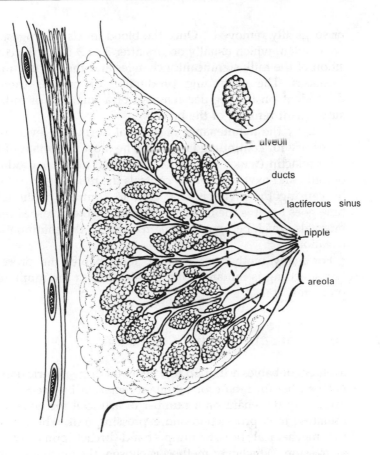

Fig. 1.1 *Anatomy of the breast. (Reproduced with permission from UNICEF.)*

plete lactation period or necessarily for that particular lactation.[25]

The shape and size of breasts differs greatly, but only rarely does this affect their primary function of providing a baby with nourishment.

1.3.1 The initiation of lactation

Lactation is possible as early as 16 weeks after conception, if the pregnancy is discontinued.[26] It is the inhibitory effects of the placental hormones, particularly progesterone, which usually delay milk production until birth and the delivery of the placenta. Indeed any fragments of retained placental material following birth can delay the onset of lactation until it is naturally or surgically removed.[26] Once the blood levels of progesterone have fallen, which usually occurs after 2 or 3 days, the composition of the milk significantly changes and the volume rapidly increases. The continuing production of milk is thereafter dependent on the regular removal of a quantity of milk and subsequent refilling of the breasts.

Initially the maintenance of optimal hormonal levels is also necessary for continuing lactation. The most important of these are prolactin (which stimulates the initial alveolar production of milk) and oxytocin (which controls the milk 'let-down' reflex by causing the myoepithelial cells to contract), although, as time goes on, it is the efficient drainage of the breast at regular intervals which becomes the main factor in the continuation of lactation.

For many mothers of healthy, term babies the process of breastfeeding is initiated and sustained with the minimum of problems.

1.3.2   Artificial stimulation of lactation

Mothers of babies admitted to a neonatal or paediatric unit may not be able to initiate or maintain lactation by breastfeeding. They may be reliant on a number of artificial methods for stimulating milk production and expressing milk. These include: the mechanical breast pump, hand breast pump or hand expression. Whichever method is chosen, the normal stimuli of breastfeeding are absent. This can have an effect on the mother's long-term chances of maintaining her milk supply and establishing exclusive breastfeeding.

The mothers' 'let-down' reflex responds to a number of different stimuli, which include touching, seeing and hearing her baby, as well as her baby's own particular scent. These stimuli may be partially or totally lacking when artificial expression is necessary. In addition, certain situations, which may condition a response before a baby feeds, such as thinking about the baby or physical closeness, may be similarly affected if a mother has to express in a setting far from her baby. Temporary inhibition of her 'let-down' response may occur when a mother is subjected to sudden and unpleasant physical or physiological stimuli, such as may be experienced on a neonatal or paediatric unit. This applies particularly when a mother is under acute stress, although minor or chronic stress does not appear to permanently affect the milk supply in the long term.[26] Nevertheless, short-term variations in the milk production can psychologically affect the mother, and if this is compounded by insufficient support from either health professionals or family members, the mother may indeed find it difficult to sustain her milk production for any prolonged period of time.

1.4   The composition and sequence of milk production

Breastmilk is a constantly changing substance, varying in composition:

- During an individual feed (i.e. fore-milk to hind-milk).
- Throughout the course of the day.[27]
- With the stage of lactation.
- Between different mothers.
- In the same mother between the two breasts and in different pregnancies.[28]
- Between preterm and term milk.[29]
- With maternal diet, which may also influence its composition.[30, 31]
- With exercise, which may have an effect by increasing the lactose content of the milk.[32]

1.4.1   Appearance of the stages of milk production

The colour of the milk is not indicative of its nutritional state. Initially colostrum is produced. This is a thick viscous fluid which can appear quite creamy in colour or more like plasma. Over the following 2 or 3 weeks the milk appears less dense and more watery as less colostrum is present. It changes gradually from a creamy white appearance to a blueish white colour.

1.4.2   The composition of breastmilk

There are three identifiable stages of lactation: production of colostrum, transitional milk and mature milk (see Fig. 1.2).

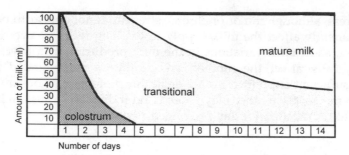

Fig. 1.2 *The sequence of milk production.*

Colostrum

Colostrum has very special properties, which gives it almost a medicinal quality, and certainly makes it an extremely valuable substance for any baby, and essential for preterm and sick babies. Its functions are still not completely understood,[33] though protection from infection is certainly one of its major roles. It is secreted in the first 3–4 days following birth. Thereafter, it gradually changes into mature milk over a 10–15-day period, during which time the milk increases in volume, and continues to change subtly in composition. Colostrum is produced in smaller quantities than mature milk – from as little as 5–10 ml at each feed or expression – but the range is considerable (5–100 ml).[34] Despite the small quantity produced, colostrum initially provides sufficient fluid and nutrients in the first few days of life for a term, healthy baby.

Colostrum is especially rich in proteins, particularly the immunoglobulins IgM, IgG and secretory IgA, and also lactoferrin and lysozymes, which together with the macrophages, lymphocytes and neutrophils (active cells) protect the newborn infant from infections – especially those to which the mother has previously been exposed and has become immune. Secretory IgA is a particularly important immunoglobulin, as it is thought to line the surface of the intestine, thereby protecting a baby from gastrointestinal infections. Another very important protein in colostrum, in concentrations five times greater than in mature milk, is epidermal growth factor (EGF),[35] known to stimulate cellular growth.[36]

Apart from its anti-infective role, colostrum also has a mild, but nevertheless an important, laxative effect, helping to clear meconium from the body and thereby preventing the reabsorption of bilirubin, which may cause jaundice in the early days of life.[37]

In some cultures it is common for colostrum not to be given to new babies. However, several studies have suggested that it is valuable not only in preventing disease in vulnerable preterm babies, but also in treating infections.[38,39] Indeed, there is evidence of its therapeutic use in Ayurvedic medicine (in the Indian sub-continent) to treat certain skin and eye infections in the general population.[40] In Japan an antibiotic 'Lactofelicine' has been developed from human colostrol proteins. This substance is claimed to be strong enough to kill the bacteria that cause food poisoning within 1 hour. Beneficial gut bacteria are left unharmed by the substance, which is active against *E. coli*, *Listeria* and other bacteria causing diarrhoea.[38] Colostrum has, therefore, a vitally important role in the initial well-being of all babies.

Mature human milk

The major constituents of breast milk are fat, protein, carbohydrate, water, vitamins, minerals and trace elements, as well as hormones, enzymes, growth factors, immunological properties and protective factors.

Fat Fat is essential for normal human development. According to one writer,[41] it forms an integral component of all cellular membranes, transports fat-soluble vitamins and hormones, and provides fatty acids which are crucial for brain development. It is also the principal source of energy in human milk, providing between 40% and 60% of the baby's total caloric intake.[42]

The fats of human milk are easily digested and absorbed by a baby, with up to 85–95% being utilized in the term baby and falling to approximately 65–80% or less in very preterm babies.[43,44]

Triglycerides are the main constituents of milk fat (98–99%).[41] These are readily broken down into free fatty acids and monoglycerides by lipases and bile salts. These lipases are present in the lingual and gastric secretions of term and preterm babies. One of the products from the breakdown process of milk fats is monolauryl, a substance with anti-bacterial, anti-viral and anti-fungal properties,[41] which may contribute to the activation of the baby's defence mechanism even before the gastric phase of digestion.

Human breastmilk itself, contains two further lipases, bile salt-stimulated lipase (BSSL) and lipoprotein lipase (LPL). BSSL is activated in the baby's small intestine,[45] where it further contributes to the digestion of fat, compensating for the low levels of pancreatic lipase and bile salt activity in newborn babies. BSSL possibly also aids improved fat absorption when a mixture of formula and the mother's own milk is given to her baby.[46] The function of the second lipase LPL in milk or in the baby is not fully understood, although it is thought to contribute to the breakdown of the triglycerides into free fatty acids and monoglycerides during storage[45,47] and is active even at 4°C.[48]

The free fatty acids in the milk have been shown to be the most important source of energy for the baby, the lipases in milk make them available even before the intestinal phase, thereby improving the energy supply. This helps to make the fat in breastmilk more easily absorbed. Pasteurization of human milk significantly reduces this absorption possibly because the milk lipases are destroyed.[49]

Breastmilk is also particularly rich in long-chain fatty acids, which have an important role in brain development and myelinization.[50] Approximately one quarter of the brain is composed of these fatty acids, of which arachidonic acid (AA) and docosahexaenoic acid (DHA) are the major components. As with many human milk factors, DHA is more concentrated in colostrum,[51] and the milk of mothers of preterm babies contains more DHA and AA than the milk of term mothers.[52]

The variability of the fat content in breastmilk   Human milk-fat content has the widest degree of variability of any milk constituent, with considerable variation between and within mothers, and during feeds.

- The lowest fat content in breastmilk is found at the beginning of a feed, in the **fore-milk**.
- The highest fat content is found towards the end of a feed in the **hind-milk**.

Opinion varies as to the exact increase in fat during the feed, but it is reported to be somewhere between double and treble.[33] Fat also varies throughout the day; some studies report that it is at its lowest in the early morning, and increases to its highest levels in early afternoon, while other studies reported the highest fat levels in the morning.[27]

Milk fat also varies with the stage of lactation. This may partly explain differences in the volume of breastmilk taken by healthy, term babies, for the total energy content of the milk may differ as the fat content varies. Therefore, it is suggested that milk with a high fat content may satisfy a baby sooner than if the fat content is low. There is even the suggestion that appetite control may develop from the different fat levels between the fore- and hind-milk.[50]

Protein Milk protein is of two types: casein and whey. Breastmilk is predominantly whey based. This forms a softer gastric curd, thereby reducing gastric emptying time and aiding digestion.[53]

Up to 90% of dietary protein can be used effectively by a baby.[53] Because absorption is efficient, less fat and protein are lost in the stools, consequently breastfed babies may pass stools less frequently than formula-fed babies.

In addition to proteins that provide nutrients, there are also anti-infective proteins. The lactoglobulin fraction of the milk contains the immunoglobulins previously mentioned in colostrum. Although these are produced in smaller quantities as the milk matures, the increased volumes of breastmilk ensure high levels of immunoglobulins are still available to the baby.[54]

Carbohydrate Lactose is the main carbohydrate in breastmilk. Small amounts of galactose, fructose and oligosaccharides are also found. Lactose provides approximately 40% of the baby's energy needs. It not only enhances the absorption of calcium and iron, but is readily broken down to galactose and glucose. Glucose provides energy to the rapidly developing brain,[33] and galactose is needed in the development of the central nervous system.[53] Lactase, the enzyme necessary in the breakdown of lactose, is present in the intestinal mucosa from birth.

In the breastfed baby, lactose encourages the growth of *Lactobacillus bifidus* in the gut. These two substances work together to keep the intestinal contents acid, thus inhibiting the growth of harmful bacteria.

The digestion of carbohydrate is helped by the enzyme amylase, which is normally found in the saliva and pancreatic juice of adults. However, it is absent in saliva at birth and in very small amounts in pancreatic juice; it is, however, present in breastmilk.

Water   Human milk is water-rich (approximately 87%). It has a low electrolyte concentration, which ensures sufficient free water is available, even when the weather is very hot or when a baby is in a tropical environment.[55]

Vitamins and minerals   The amounts of the fat-soluble vitamins A, D, E and K may vary in breastmilk according to its total fat content. Variations may similarly occur in the water-soluble vitamins, vitamin C, vitamin B complex and folic acid. Mothers who are vegans are at particular risk of vitamin deficiency, as well as mothers who are long-term users of oral contraceptives, who may have a deficiency of vitamin B_6.[56]

Vitamin K, which is important in the blood-clotting mechanism, is known to be present in higher quantities in both colostrum and hind-milk.[56] **All** babies, and certainly preterm and sick babies, should, therefore, receive both. This emphasizes the need to ensure that mothers, who need to express, begin as early as possible after birth. Breastmilk is considered to contain insufficient vitamin K for the newborn, term baby during the first few days of life until he can produce his own. Insufficient vitamin K has been associated with haemorrhagic disease of the newborn. Studies appear to indicate that there is an increased risk of this condition in babies who are breastfed compared to those who are formula fed.[57] Therefore, shortly after birth and with the parents' consent, prophylactic vitamin K is administered to all babies, either orally or by intramuscular injection, regardless of whether they are to be breast or formula fed. Extra doses may also be considered necessary for the sick and preterm baby. In the case of breastfed babies, the British Paediatric Association recommends further oral doses, either weekly or monthly for up to 26 weeks post-delivery, with no further vitamin K considered necessary for formula-fed infants after the initial dose.[58]

Although rare, vitamin D deficiency in a baby may result in neonatal rickets.[59] This may be a problem, particularly if pregnant or breastfeeding women are deficient in vitamin D themselves.[60] Babies most at risk of neonatal rickets are low birthweight or preterm and dark-skinned babies living in temperate climates where there may be little sunshine, especially during the winter months.[53] Supplements of calciferol (vitamin D) are, therefore, commonly given to these babies when they receive breastmilk.

The levels of sodium, calcium, phosphorus and magnesium

in breastmilk are considered ideal for the term, breastfed baby. However, this may not be the case for preterm babies (even though preterm breastmilk contains higher levels of these minerals). This is because of immaturity of their gastric and renal systems, particularly in babies born before 32 weeks gestation. Mineral supplementation of breastmilk to correct any deficiencies may be necessary. The manual expression of breastmilk (when expression is necessary) may be important in this context, for there is some evidence to suggest that this method of expression results in higher levels of some minerals, e.g. sodium.[61]

It has been suggested that, while breastmilk may contain significantly lower concentrations of minerals than formula milk, absorption may be enhanced in breastfed babies by the presence of specific transport factors in breastmilk.

Trace elements Iron is present in breastmilk in small amounts. A term baby, however, usually has sufficient stores of iron for at least the first 4–6 months, and may not require any supplements until solids are introduced.[62] The high levels of lactose and vitamin C in breastmilk help to facilitate iron absorption. The preterm baby, by contrast, may require iron supplementation because he is unable to absorb it effectively and breastmilk may contain insufficient amounts for his needs.

Zinc is the most abundant trace mineral in human milk; its content is approximately eight times higher in colostrum than in mature milk, with a gradual decline as lactation progresses. Because it is important to growth, it is suggested that the higher levels in the early weeks of lactation reflect the higher growth velocity during this period.[63] Zinc is also essential to enzyme structure and function, and cellular immunity.

1.5   The development of a baby's feeding ability

The ability of a baby to feed efficiently depends upon the coordination of his suck, swallow and breathing reflexes. The development of these reflexes begins during the fetal period and reaches maturity at approximately 40 weeks gestation. Therefore, a term baby is usually well able to breastfeed very soon after birth, while a preterm baby may take several days or weeks before this is possible. The question, to which there is still no really satisfactory answer, is, what kind of stimuli is most appropriate for a preterm baby, to help him learn to feed orally once outside the womb and which will also enhance the natural maturation process?

The following 'milestones' in the maturation process influence the decision of which method of feeding is the most appropriate when a baby is preterm at birth:

- Oesophageal peristalsis and swallowing have been observed in the fetus from as early as 11 weeks *in utero*.[64]
- Sucking has been observed in various studies to begin between 18 and 24 weeks.[65]
- Lingual and gastric lipases are detectable in the fetus from approximately 26 weeks gestation.[43]
- The gag reflex is evident from 26 to 27 weeks in prematurely delivered babies.[65]
- Rooting, the response shown by a baby when touching the side of his cheek to encourage him to turn to the breast, with his mouth widely open. This occurs around 32 weeks post-conception age.[65]
- A co-ordinated and effective use of the suck, swallow and breathing reflexes for nutritive purposes occurs at approximately 32–35 weeks post-conception age.
- A normal baby born at term, who is healthy, has a sufficiently mature suck and swallow reflex to breastfeed within a very short time of birth.[66]

Therefore, up to 30 weeks gestation or post-conception age, a baby is unlikely to be fed orally. Most of his milk feeds will be given by gastric tube (and he may also require intravenous fluids). Some well preterm babies as young as 28 weeks are able to lick the milk expressed on to the nipple by the mother. From approximately 30 weeks in some babies, small amounts of oral feeding are possible. Between 30 and 32 weeks, breastmilk can be given by cup or can be expressed directly into a baby's mouth, and he will be able to lick milk from the nipple. Some babies may be able to attach at the breast although they may not yet begin to suckle, while others may suckle quite vigorously considering how young they are. For the majority of babies at this age, breastmilk will still be given mainly by gastric tube.

From 32 to 34 weeks gestation or post-conception age, gastric tube feeding may still be important, but some babies will be able to take a complete breastfeed on one or several occasions over a 24-hour period. Most babies at this age will be able to cup-feed well and take appropriate amounts of fluid by this method. From 35 weeks onward, efficient breastfeeding is possible, and by 37 weeks gestation or post-conception age a well baby is usually able to sustain his nutrition totally at the breast.

1.6 Factors affecting a baby's ability to feed efficiently

A number of conditions may affect a baby's ability to feed efficiently. These may be may be physical, neurological, chromosomal, metabolic or clinical in origin.

Physical problems which affect the mechanics of feeding include:

- Cleft lip and/or palate.
- A very high curved palate, which can occur in preterm babies who have been ventilated for a long period of time (although oral plates may prevent or reduce the likelihood of this occurring).
- A short frenulum to the tongue (tongue tie).
- A protruding or large tongue, which is a feature in some babies with Down's syndrome.
- A small and receding lower jaw and a short tongue, as in Pierre Robin syndrome.

Other physical conditions that do not affect the baby's ability to feed orally but affect the overall efficiency of feeding, include pyloric stenosis (causing a narrowing of the muscular wall of the pylorus between the stomach and the jejunem).

While there is no doubt that some of the above conditions may interfere with efficient oral feeding, breastfeeding may be easier to establish and more successful than bottle feeding. If a mother has an efficient 'let-down' reflex, the baby may be able to obtain sufficient quantities of milk without having to expend a lot of energy or physical effort.

The co-ordination of the suck, swallow and breathing reflexes may be compromised by extreme prematurity or illness (causing a baby to be weak). For apparently healthy babies of 36+ weeks gestation or post-conception age whose reflexes do not appear to be well co-ordinated, the reasons may be difficult to identify. These babies are commonly among those admitted to neonatal or paediatric units with 'feeding problems' within the first few days after delivery. One explanation may be that some term babies naturally take several days to develop a mature sucking pattern and that it is not uncommon for a 1–2 day period to elapse before a mature pattern emerges. It also appears that the lower the gestational age of the baby, the longer the period required to develop a mature pattern of sucking, so that it may take a baby of 32 weeks up to 6–8 weeks to show a mature pattern.[67]

Maternal analgesia or sedation used during labour may affect a baby's readiness to feed, and his level of arousal. Pethidine has certainly been implicated in babies failing to feed efficiently in the first few days after birth.[68]

Babies with a neurological condition frequently have problems co-ordinating their suck, swallow and breathing reflexes. They may have a number of symptoms,[69] which interfere with their ability to feed by any conventional method. These include:

- A weak suck, swallow and gag reflex.
- A tongue movement that is abnormal.
- A sucking movement that shows no regular pattern.
- An abnormal 'biting' action.
- Flaccid muscle tone of the mouth and head (and of the whole body).
- Excessive arching of the body.

Babies with respiratory and cardiac problems tire easily, and use more calories to maintain respiration and circulation. They usually gain weight slowly regardless of how they are fed. Increasing the volume of breastmilk to ensure adequate nutrient and calorie content may not be possible because the volume required may be too great or, during the acute or chronic phase of the baby's condition, they may be fluid restricted and need a nutrient/calorie-dense supplement.

The mother's 'natural' nipple shape may affect a baby's attachment at the breast. Flat or inverted nipples, for example, may be more difficult for a preterm or weak baby to draw effectively into his mouth to form a 'long teat' of breast tissue. A long nipple, by contrast, may make correct attachment difficult to achieve. A baby, particularly if he is preterm, may not be able to reach the lactiferous sinuses during the suckling action. Attention to attachment and positioning is critical in this situation.

Certain metabolic disorders may make breastfeeding and the use of expressed breastmilk impossible. These include very rare conditions in which there is a primary deficiency of lactase, the enzyme vital in the breakdown of lactose. Galactosaemia, for example, also affects the metabolism of lactose, because the liver enzyme galactose is missing. Such conditions become very obvious in the first weeks of life but fortunately are very uncommon.

References

1 Williams AF (1993) Human milk and the preterm baby. Lancet **306**: 1628–1629.
2 Helsing E and King FS (1982) Breast-feeding in Practice: A Manual for Health Workers. Oxford: Oxford University Press, Ch. 19, p. 178.
3 World Health Organization (1984) Infant feeding: the physiological basis. Bulletin (Suppl.) **67**: 30–31.
4 World Health Organization (1993) Global breast-feeding prevalence and trends. In Breast-feeding: The Technical Basis and Recommendations for Action. Saadch RJ, Labock MH, Cooney KA, Koniz-Booher P (eds). Geneva: WHO, pp. 1–19.
5 Lucas A and Cole TJ (1990) Breast milk and necrotising enterocolitis. Lancet **336**: 1519–1523.
6 Howie PJ, Forsyth J, Ogston SA, et al. Protective effect of breast feeding against infection. Br Med J **300**: 11–16.
7 Labbock MH and Henderson GE (1987) Does breastfeeding protect against malocclusion? Am J Prev **3**: 227.
8 Saarinen UM (1982) Prolonged breastfeeding as prophylaxis for recurrent otitis media. Acta Pediatr Scand **3**: 227–232.
9 Williamson IG, Dunleavey J and Robinson D (1994) Risk factors in otitis media with effusion. A 1 year case control study in 5–7 year old children. Family Practice **11**: 271–274.
10 Park P (1992) Cows' milk linked to juvenile diabetes. New Scientist **1835**: 9 (22 August).
11 Karjalainen I, Martin JM, Knip M, Ilonen J, Robinson BH, Savilahati E, Akerblom HK and Dosch H-M (1992) A bovine albumin peptide as a possible trigger of insulin-dependent diabetes mellitus. New Engl J Med **327**: 302–307.
12 Lucas A, Morley R, Cole TJ, Lister G and Leeson-Payne C (1992) Breast milk and subsequent intelligence quotient in children born preterm. Lancet **339**: 261–264.
13 Farquharson J, Cockburn F, Patrick WA, Jamison EC and Logan RW (1992) Infant cerebral cortex phospholipid fatty-acid composition and diet. Lancet **340**: 810–813.
14 Lucas A and Cole TJ (1990) Breast milk and neonatal necrotising enterocolitis. Lancet **336**: 1519–1521.
15 Shu XO, Clemens J, Zheng W, Ying DM, Ji BT and Jin F (1995)

Infant breastfeeding and the risk of childhood lymphoma and leukemia. *Int J Epidemiol* **24**: 27–32.

16 Matthew DJ, Taylor B, Norman AP, Turner MW and Soothill JF (1977) Prevention of eczema. *Lancet* **1**: 321–324.

17 Newcomb PA, Storer BE, Longnecker MP, Mittendorf R, Greenberg ER, Clapp RW, Burke KP, Willett WC and MacMahon B (1994) Lactation and a reduced risk of premenopausal breast cancer. *New Engl J Med*, **330**: 81–87.

18 Reuter K, Baker SP and Krolikowski FJ (1992) Risk factors for breast cancer in women undergoing mammography. *Am J Roentgenol* **158**: 273–278.

19 Yoo KY, Tajima K, Kuroishi T, Hirose K, Yoshida M, Miura S and Murai H (1992) Independent protective effect of lactation against breast cancer: A case-control study in Japan. *Am J Epidemiol* **135**: 726–733.

20 Cummings RG and Klineberg RJ (1993) Breastfeeding and other reproductive factors and the risk of hip fracture in elderly women. *Int J Epidemiol* **2**: 684–691.

21 Gross B (1991) Is the lactational amenorrhea method a part of natural family planning? Biology and policy. *Am J Obstet Gynecol* **165**: 2014–2019.

22 Lewis PR, Brown JB, Renfree MB and Short RV (1991) The resumption of ovulation and menstruation in a well-nourished population of women breastfeeding for an extended period of time. *Fertil Steril* **55**: 529–536.

23 Dugdale AE and Eaton-Evans J (1989) The effect of lactation and other factors on post-partum changes in body-weight and triceps skinfold thickness. *Br J Nutrition* **61**: 149–153.

24 World Health Organization (1993) *Breastfeeding: The Technical Basis and Recommendations for Action.* Saadeh RJ (ed.) Geneva: World Health Organization.

25 World Health Organization (1989) Infant Feeding: the physiological basis. *Bulletin* (Suppl.) **67**: 20.

26 World Health Organization (1989) Infant feeding: the physiological basis. *Bulletin* (Suppl.) **67**: 21.

27 Lammi-Keefe CJ, Ferris AM and Jensen RG (1990) Changes in human milk at 0600, 1000, 1400, 1800, and 2200 h. *J Pediatr Gastroent Nut* **11**: 83–88.

28 Burman D (1982) Nutrition in early childhood. In Nutrition in growth and development, Part I. *Textbook of Paediatric Nutrition*, 2nd edn. McLaren D, Burman D (eds). Edinburgh: Churchill Livingstone, pp. 39–72.

29 Gross SJ, David RJ, Bauman L and Tomarelli RM (1980) Nutritional composition of milk produced by mothers delivering preterm. *J Pediatics* **96**: 641–644.

30 Silber GH, Hachey DL, Schanler RJ and Garza C (1988) Manipulation of maternal diet to alter fatty acid composition of human milk intended for premature infants. *Am J Clin Nutrition* **47**: 810–814.

31 Specker BL (1994) Nutritional concerns of lactating women con-

suming vegetarian diets. *Am J Clin Nutrition* **59**(Suppl.): 1182S–1186S.

32 Wallace JP, Inbar G and Ernsthausen K (1992) Infant acceptance of postexercise breast milk. *Pediatrics* **89**: 1245–1247.

33 Jelliffe DB and Jelliffe EFP (1978) Biochemical considerations. *Human Milk in the Modern World*. Oxford: Oxford University Press, p. 28.

34 Odent M (1990) The unknown human infant. *J Human Lact* **6**: 6–8.

35 Jannson L, Karlson FA and Westermark D (1985) Mitogenic activity and epidermal growth factor content in human milk. *Acta Paeditr Scand* **74**: 250–253.

36 Carpenter G (1980) Epidermal growth factor is a major growth-promoting agent in human milk. *Science* **210**: 198–199.

37 De Carvalho M, Klaus MH and Merkatz RB (1982) Frequency of breast-feeding and serum bilirubin. *Am J Dis Child* **136**: 737–738.

38 Cure in a mother's milk. *New Scientist* 20 April 1991.

39 Mathur NB, Dwarkadas AM, Sharma VK, Saha K and Jain N (1990) Anti-infective factors in preterm human colostrum. *Acta Paediatr Scand* **79**: 1039–1044.

40 Reissland N and Burghart R (1988) The quality of a mothers milk and the health of her child: beliefs and practices of the women of Mithila. *Social Sci Med* **27**: 461–469.

41 Hamosh M, Bitman J, Fink CS, Freed LM, York CM, Wood DL, Mehta NR and Hamosh P (1985) Lipid composition of preterm human milk and its digestion by the infant. In *Composition and Physiological Properties of Human Milk*. Schaub J (ed.). Oxford: Elsevier Science Publishers, pp. 153–164.

42 Steichen JJ, Krug-Wispe SK and Tsang RC (1987) Breastfeeding the low birth weight infant. *Clinics Perinatol* **14**: 1.

43 Hamosh M (1987) Lipid metabolism in premature infants. *Biol Neonate* **52** (Suppl.): 50–64.

44 Hamosh M (1979) A review. Fat digestion in the newborn: role of lingual lipase and preduodenal digestion. *Pediatr Res* **13**: 615–622.

45 Hernell O and Blackberg L (1988) Lipolysis in human milk: causes and consequences. In *Composition and Physiological Properties of Human Milk*. Schaub J (ed.). Oxford: Elsevier Science Publishers, pp. 165–178.

46 Hamosh M, Bitman J, Fink CS, Freed LM, York CM, Wood DL, Mehta NR and Hamosh P (1985) Lipid composition of preterm human milk and its digestion by the infant. In *Composition and Physiological Properties of Human Milk*. Schaub J (ed.). Oxford: Elsevier Science Publishers, pp. 153–162.

47 Freed LM, Neville MC and Hamosh M (1986) Diurnal and within-feed variations in lipase activity and triglyceride content of human milk. *J Pediatr Gastroenterol Nutrition* **5**: 938–942.

48 Jelliffe DB and Jelliffe EFP (1978) Biochemical considerations. *Human Milk in the Modern World*. Oxford: Oxford University Press, p. 28.

49 Canadian Paediatric Society: Committee on Nutrition (1981) Feeding the low birth weight infant. *Can Med Assoc* **124**: 1301–1311.

50   Jackson KA and Gibson RA (1989) Weaning foods cannot replace breast milk as sources of long-chain polyunsaturated fatty acids. *Am J Clin Nutrition* **50**: 980–982.

51   Nettleton JA (1993) Are n-3 fatty acids essential nutrients for fetal and infant development? *J Am Diet Assoc* **93**: 58–64.

52   Ghebremeskel K and Leighfield M (1992) Infant brain lipids and diet (letter). *Lancet* **340**: 1093.

53   World Health Organization (1989) Infant feeding: the physiological basis. *Bulletin* **67** (Suppl.): 25–26.

54   Jatsyk GV, Kuvaeva IB and Gribakin SG (1985) Immunological protection of the neonatal gastrointestinal tract: the importance of breastfeeding. *Acta Paediatr Scand* **74**: 246–249.

55   Almroth S and Bidinger PD (1990) No need for water supplementation for exclusively breast-fed infants under hot and arid conditions. *Trans Roy Soc Trop Med Hygiene* **84**: 602–604.

56   World Health Organization (1989) Infant feeding: the physiological basis. *Bulletin* **67** (Suppl.): 28–29.

57   McNinch AW and Tripp JH (1991) Haemorrhagic disease of the newborn in the British Isles: two-year prospective study. *Br Med J* **303**: 1105–1109.

58   British Paediatric Association (1992) *Vitamin K Prophylaxis in Infancy. Report of an Expert Committee.* London: British Paediatric Association.

59   Chang YT, Germain-Lee EL, Doran TF, Migeon CJ, Levine MA and Berkowitz GD (1992) Hypocalcaemia in non-white breast-fed infants. *Clin Pediatr* **31**: 695–698.

60   Rothberg AD, Pettifor JM, Cohen DF, Sonnendecker EWW and Ross PF (1982) Maternal–infant vitamin D relationships during breast-feeding. *J Pediatr* **101**: 500–503.

61   Lang S, Lawrence CJ and L'E Orme R (1994) Sodium in hand and pump expressed human breast milk. *Early Hum Dev* **38**: 131–138.

62   DHSS (1991) *Present Day Practice in Infant Feeding: Third Report,* 4th edn. London: HMSO.

63   Riordan J (1993) The biologic specificity of breastmilk. In *Breastfeeding and Human Lactation.* Riordan J, Auerbach KG (eds). London, Jones & Bartlett, pp. 105–129.

64   Lebenthal E, Heitlinger L, Milla PJ (1988) Prenatal and perinatal development of the gastrointestinal tract. In *Harries Paediatric Gastroenterology,* 2nd edn, Milla PJ, Muller DPR (eds). Edinburgh: Churchill Livingstone.

65   McBride MC and Danner SC (1987) Sucking disorders in neurologically impaired infants: assessment and facilitation of breastfeeding. *Clinics Perinatol* **14**: 109–130.

66   Widstrom A-M and Thingstrom-Pausson J (1993) The position of the tongue during rooting reflexes elicited in newborn infants before the first suckle. *Acta Paediatr Scand* **82**: 281–283.

67   Meyer Palmer M, Crawley K and Blanco IA (1993) Neonatal oral-motor assessment scale: a reliability study. *J Perinatol* **8**: 30–35.

68   Righard L and Alade MO (1990) Effect of delivery room routines on success of first breast-feed. *Lancet* **336**: 1105–1107.

69   La Leche League International (1992). The neurologically impaired baby. *The Breastfeeding Answer Book,* Vol. 15, pp. 336–337.

2 The position and attachment of the baby at the breast

2.1 Positioning and breast attachment

This chapter is primarily concerned with the positioning and breast attachment of babies who have special needs, i.e. they may be small, have low energy reserves, be clinically unwell, or have temporarily or permanently impaired oral function.

For these babies, many of whom will be in a neonatal or paediatric unit, an imaginative and flexible approach is essential. It may be that for the majority of mothers and babies in these units the more common breastfeeding positions are ideal. However, where this is not the case it is worth experimenting to find a position which will work for the mother and her baby – even if it needs to be changed at a later date or looks a bit strange! The important point is for the mother and baby to be content, and succeed in breastfeeding in a way which suits their individual needs. At the same time it should be borne in mind that the baby's position and attachment at the breast are crucial not only to the success of breastfeeding but also to the maintenance of healthy breasts and nipples.

2.1.1 Positioning, monitoring and oxygen therapy

Many of the babies in a neonatal or specialist paediatric unit are likely to require some form of monitoring – measuring heart rate, respiration or oxygen saturation. In most cases this involves a cable between the monitoring apparatus and the baby. Breastfeeding a baby attached to a large monitor should **not** be a problem as long as the mother's chair is close enough to the monitor to ensure that all connections are secure.

Small portable monitors, measuring respirations, can easily

be tucked into the blanket or sheet used to wrap the baby, or else they can simply be placed in the mother's lap. Often the small respiration monitors can be disconnected while the baby is being held by the mother.

A baby receiving oxygen should also have no problems breastfeeding, as long as the oxygen requirement is not so high as to necessitate the baby receiving it via a headbox. A funnel placed over the mother's shoulder, near the baby's face, should be adequate if the baby does not have nasal cannulae. As with monitor cables, it is important to be sure the mother's chair is close enough to the source of oxygen and that any tubes are long enough, without being pulled taut when the mother and baby are comfortably positioned in a chair.

2.1.2   Before positioning and attaching the baby at the breast

1. Ensure privacy, particularly in the initial period while the mother and baby are learning what to do. This may be achieved simply by using screens, or even by turning the mother's chair away from other people in a quiet part of a unit or a room set aside for this purpose. Conversely, breastfeeding should not be something a mother feels she has to 'go away' and do in private. She should feel that she can feed discretely anywhere she chooses. Therefore, what she wears, and how confident she is in her feeding skills are very important. A neonatal unit can be a very positive 'training' environment for a mother to feed in, giving her time to become comfortable with breastfeeding when other people are around.
2. The mother needs to be sitting comfortably.

   (a) If the mother is in a chair, it should:
      - Be wide enough for both the mother and baby to be comfortable.
      - Be low enough for the mother's feet to be flat on the floor.
      - Have arm rests on which the mother can support **her** arms; this helps her to support her baby (see Fig. 2.1).

Whilst a rocking chair may be comfortable and relaxing once

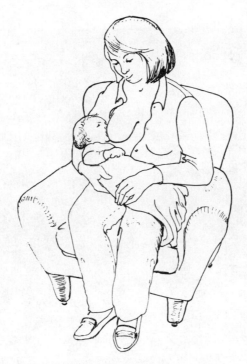

Fig. 2.1 *An ideal nursing chair.*

the establishment of breastfeeding has taken place, it may not provide enough stability for the mother and baby while they are learning to breastfeed.

   (b) If the mother is on a bed or on the floor:
- She will require sufficient pillows around her for firm comfortable support.
- She may find a soft pillow placed under her knees adds to her comfort.

3.   The mother's clothing should be practical, for example, blouses or dresses with buttons down the front, or loose, T-shirt style tops. A hair clip, 'bulldog' clip or a peg are useful for holding clothing away from the mother's breast, so that she does not have to support her clothes with her hand (see Fig. 2.2). The brassiere or upper garment must not be tight around the margins of the breast or restrict access to the nipple area, as this may prevent efficient drainage of the milk, resulting in a blocked duct or lobe.

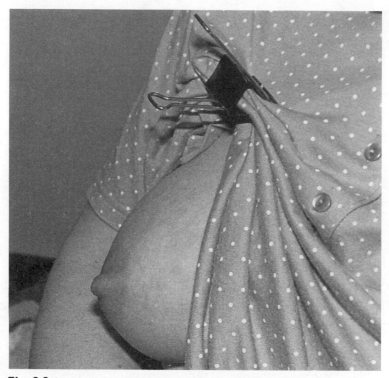

Fig. 2.2 *A method of securing clothing to make breastfeeding easier.*

4. A preterm baby – particularly one less than 35 weeks – may benefit from being lightly wrapped for a breastfeed. This reduces the amount of stimulation received through moving his arms, which may distract him from his feeding experience. A term baby does not need to be wrapped up to breastfeed, though some mothers may find it easier to feed when the baby's arms are not in the way. However, it is not unusual to observe a term healthy baby touch or stroke his mother's breasts before or during a feed. Although it has not been fully researched, it may be beneficial for the baby to do this. If the nipple is touched it may be stimulated to become more erect and thus enhance attachment. In addition, though not necessarily physiologically related, the tactile stimulation of the baby fingering the mother's nipple and areola may encourage the release of the hormones prolactin and oxytocin and thereby, aid an efficient milk flow.

5. **Small** blankets, towels and soft pillows should be available to support the baby; these can be positioned easily by the mother without help. They need to be on a table or stool placed near enough to the mother to be within easy reach of her. Larger pillows can be too bulky for this purpose and are more difficult for the mother to position herself when she is on her own.

6. A drink should be available within easy reach of the mother! **Beware** of very hot fluids – they can cause burns.

Finally, it is important to have **time** to help a mother and, if helping her practically, that you too are sitting comfortably on a small chair or stool. Do not stoop to help her for **you** risk damaging **your** back.

2.1.3 Positions for breastfeeding

There are several positions in which a mother can breastfeed her baby. Initially, it is important for the mother to find a position which she finds comfortable and is therefore most likely to lead to successful breastfeeding. Equally, it is essential for the mother to have her baby positioned in such a way that she is in control of attaching the baby to the breast herself and does not depend upon the help of a second person.

The mother may have definite views about which position she wishes to use (especially if she has breastfed before). However, for a baby compromised by size or clinical condition, positions which are appropriate in the early days of feeding may be new to the mother and it is important to explain why a different position may be more appropriate until the baby is older and bigger.

It is therefore useful to teach a mother more than one position for breastfeeding. Alternative positions may be appropriate in a number of different situations – for example, as small babies grow bigger and stronger; to give a mother flexibility if she is using an unconventional breastfeeding position at home (for any reason) but wishes to use a more conventional position when she goes out; and for babies pre- and post-surgery who have a cleft lip and palate. In addition, a baby's position at the breast may have direct influence on how effectively he is attached and, therefore, how effectively he drains the whole breast rather than only part of it. Hence, mothers who experience blocked lobes or mastitis may find that using another position for breastfinding facilitates an improved attachment at the breast, thus achieving better drainage.

The 'underarm' position

The underarm position is ideal for small and preterm babies (and larger ones too!) (Fig. 2.3).

The advantages of this position are:

- When a baby has a 'small' mouth, and the nipple and areola appear impossibly large, attachment is easier in this position.
- It enables a mother to see the position of her baby's tongue, which must be in the floor of the mouth prior to attachment.
- It is a comfortable and secure way of holding a baby and at the same time the mother has a completely free hand.
- It is useful at bath times for washing the baby's hair.

An easy way to teach the mother this position so that she will be comfortable is to help her to position her baby while she is standing. The baby should be held in a supine position with his lower body tucked into the mother's waist, just above her hip. The mother, using the arm on the same side of her

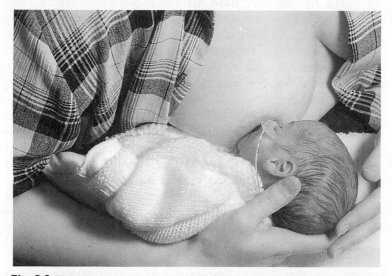

Fig. 2.3 The underarm position for breastfeeding. (Photo courtesy of the North Staffs Neonatal Unit and Egnell-Ameda.)

body as the baby is positioned, supports the baby's head with her hand and uses the length of her forearm to support the full length of his body. When she then sits down her body is straight and she is more relaxed as a result. When the baby is positioned with the mother already sitting, she often unconsciously leans towards her baby and very quickly becomes tired and uncomfortable.

To help the mother gain confidence in handling her baby, when she is standing up and has the baby positioned, encourage her to take him for a small walk around the area of the cot or incubator. Even if the baby is attached to an array of monitors, the mother can take a few steps with him in the underarm position. (If the baby is very fragile, it is best to walk with him when his condition is more stable.)

How to attach a baby in the underarm position to the breast The mother should 'cup' the baby's head in her hand rather than grip the back of the head, which may be painful and cause the baby to be irritable and pull away from the breast. Alternatively, the mother can support the base of her baby's head between her thumb and fingers (Fig. 2.3). Supporting the baby's head gives the mother maximum control and enables her to slightly extend her baby's head, making it easier for him to suckle effectively. The mother may offer her baby the breast by positioning her four fingers under the breast and use her thumb and forefinger to position and shape the nipple (using the same positioning as for hand expression). In this position it is easy to touch and lightly brush the baby's mouth or cheek with the nipple, to encourage rooting, that is, the baby turning his head towards the breast with his mouth opened widely (Fig. 2.4). At this point the mother should move the baby quickly on to the breast. Once the baby is correctly attached, the mother can take her fingers away from the breast.

A modification of this position is useful if a baby needs to be fed while laying flat. This may arise if the baby is wearing a plaster splint or has had abdominal surgery, or has an oral defect – such as a cleft lip and palate (unilateral or bilateral), where it may be an advantage if the areola and nipple 'fall' directly into the baby's mouth. The baby should be positioned with his lower body and legs supported on a pillow which is as high as the mother's lap, so that he can remain flat. The mother does not need to support his body with her forearm, but she should support his head in her hand. The baby should

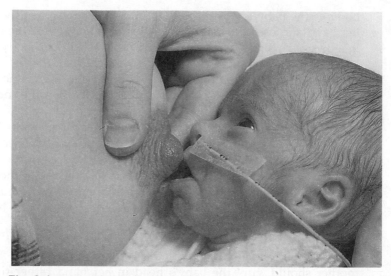

Fig. 2.4. *Encouraging a preterm baby to open his mouth. (Photo courtesy of the North Staffs Neonatal Unit and Egnell-Ameda.)*

be in a position where she can easily lean forward and let her breast fall into his mouth. She may require a second person to help adjust the position of the baby so that his whole body is aligned.

The mother may find it helps to have a table in front of her with a comfortable pillow to lean her head on so that she does not become tired or stiff. The advantage of this position is that she has one hand free to help with attachment or to express milk directly into her baby's mouth.

The 'traditional' position

The traditional position is useful for a larger baby (Fig. 2.5). The mother can either support the baby's head on her forearm or with the hand opposite the breast from which the baby will feed. A term baby who is able to breastfeed with no difficulty may have no problem with her head being supported on the forearm, but it may initially help a mother learn to attach her baby to the breast if she supports the baby's head with her hand, as this gives her more control of the head. If the baby's head is supported in the crook of the mother's elbow, the baby will be too far to the side for the mother to feed him comfortably for any length of time.

A baby who 'prefers' one side will often take both sides, if

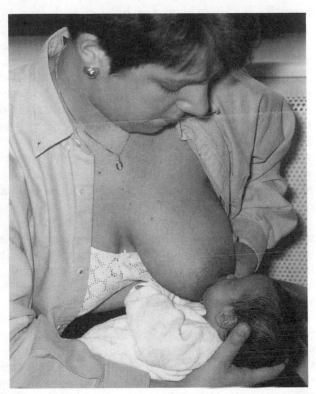

Fig. 2.5 *The 'traditional' position for breastfeeding. (Photo courtesy of the North Staffs Neonatal Unit and Egnell-Ameda.)*

held in the traditional position for the preferred side and the underarm position for the other side.

Other useful positions

Laying down with the baby alongside is a useful position for:

- A mother who has had a Caesarean section.
- A baby who has a cleft lip/and or palate.
- A baby who has poor head control.
- A mother who is disabled and cannot take the weight of the baby in her arms.

A mother who is unable to sit up can feed her baby while laying on her back if the baby is placed on her chest. She will need help to position the baby across her chest.

Breastfeeding more than one baby at each feed

A combination of positions can be used by mothers feeding more than one baby at the same time. Twins, for example, can be held with both in the 'underarm' positions – one on each side, or both in the traditional position. Alternatively, one twin can be held in the 'traditional' position and one in the 'underarm' position. Whichever position the mother is most comfortable in and can manage herself should be used. A 'V'-shaped pillow placed around her with the 'V' at the front may help in supporting the twins. These positions are also suitable for mothers 'tandem' feeding, i.e. feeding a newborn baby and an older child at the same time.

The mother may experience initial difficulties with positioning two babies at the breast at the same time – and in trying to get comfortable herself. She may find to begin with that it is easier to position her babies and even feed them separately. Once they are fed and settled she can try experimenting with different ways of holding them together.

Twins commonly feed from only one breast each. This is not normally a problem, for each breast is quite able to provide sufficient milk for their needs. However, if one twin is bigger than the other, or if one twin gains weight more quickly than the other, it may help to swap them to feed from the opposite breasts (i.e. the breast they do not usually feed from). In this way the breasts are both stimulated to produce adequate amounts of milk.

2.1.4   Breast attachment

For a baby to breastfeed successfully he has to be able to drain the lactiferous sinuses. The baby must therefore, take much of the areola into his mouth. To do this the baby forms a long 'teat' from the breast tissue,[1] with the nipple forming approximately one-third of this 'teat'. The baby's tongue is to the front of his mouth and positioned over his lower gums, beneath the lactiferous sinuses. It is 'cupped' round the 'teat' of breast tissue. The tongue moves in a 'wave'-like action from the front to the back. This 'wave' causes the 'teat' of breast tissue to be pressed against the hard palate, which squeezes the milk out of the lactiferous sinuses into the baby's mouth (see Fig. 2.6).

The baby does not 'suck' the milk out of the breast. Suction

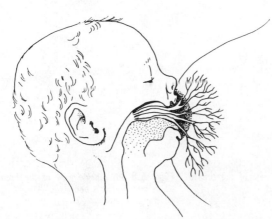

Fig. 2.6 *An inside view of the breast, when attachment is good.*

helps to form the long 'teat' and then to hold the breast tissue in the baby's mouth. The milk is removed by rhythmic compression and release of the lactiferous sinuses.

To attach a baby correctly:

1. The baby's head and body should be in a straight line.
2. His face should face the breast with his nose or upper lip opposite the mother's nipple.
3. The baby should be encouraged to open his mouth widely (by touching his cheek or lips with a finger or nipple).
4. Once the baby opens his mouth widely he needs to be moved quickly on to the breast.
5. The baby's lower lip should be aimed below the mother's nipple so that his chin touches the breast. A possible exception to this may be when positioning and attaching a baby with a small lower jaw, such as in Pierre Robin Syndrome. Then the baby's chin should be as close to the mother's breast as possible. More of the mother's areola should be visible above the baby's mouth than below (Fig. 2.7).

If the baby is poorly attached (Fig. 2.8) the following signs are likely to be seen:[1]

- The baby's chin does not touch the mother's breast.

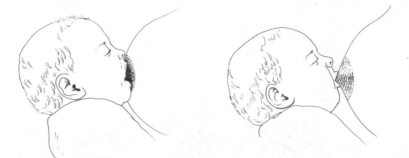

Fig. 2.7 *An outside view of the breast when attachment is good.*   **Fig. 2.8** *An outside view of the breast when attachment is poor.*

- The baby's mouth is not wide open and his lips may be almost closed.
- The baby's lower lip is not turned outwards, instead his lips are pursed forwards.
- The same amount of areola can be seen above and below the baby's mouth.

The results of poor attachment include:

- Breast engorgement.
- Sore or cracked nipples.
- An unsettled baby because the milk is not flowing quickly enough.
- A baby who wants to feed very often or for very long periods.
- A baby who refuses to feed, gains weight very slowly or who begins to lose weight.

2.1.5 How to remove a baby from the breast

If for any reason a mother needs to take her baby off the breast before a feed is finished, or because the baby has not attached to the breast comfortably, the easiest and most effective way is for the mother to insert her little finger into the side of the baby's mouth to break the seal around the breast tissue, and then gently remove the baby from the breast.

Sore or damaged nipples and areola can result from 'pulling' the baby from the breast before the seal around the tissues has been broken.

2.1.6 How to help a baby with difficulty attaching to the breast

Some babies have difficulty becoming attached to the breast because they have very low energy levels, or have a specific weakness of the muscles involved in feeding caused by a neurological or chromosomal abnormality. If this weakness affects their lower jaw, the following position may be of some use.

The baby's attachment at the breast can be helped by the mother supporting both her breast and her baby's chin at the same time. In this way, the mother is able to assist the baby to maintain his attachment, so that when he pauses or becomes tired his lower jaw does not fall away from the breast and affect his attachment. This position for attachment is known as the 'Dancer' position (see Fig. 2.9).

To use this technique the mother should:

1. Position the baby comfortably at the breast in an upright sitting position.
2. Make sure the baby is well supported (use small blankets, towels if necessary) and the hand opposite the breast is free.
3. Place her thumb and first finger on either side of the baby's chin.

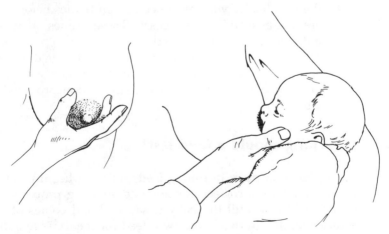

Fig. 2.9 *The 'Dancer' position for attachment at the breast.*

4.   Place the other three fingers under the breast.
5.   When the baby opens his mouth and is attached to the breast, continue to support his head and chin as described.

2.1.7   How to attach a baby to the breast who has become used to a bottle teat or dummy

Both a dummy and a teat of a bottle provide a hard, unyielding and constant stimulus to the area between the hard and soft palate. This stimulates the baby to suck. If the baby becomes used to this stimuli attachment at the breast may be more difficult. This is because the nipple and areola of the breast are softer and produce a more subtle form of palate stimulation. However, it may be useful if a mother gently massages the nipple for a few seconds just before attachment, so that it becomes hard or more erect, and then follows the steps to attachment given in Section 2.1.4. Slight pressure from the mother's forefinger or thumb on the areola (approximately 2.5 cm   from the nipple) usually results in the nipple facing slightly upwards. If this is done at the time of attachment it may help the 'hardened' nipple to come into contact with the palate and thus initiate a sucking response.

Babies who may benefit from this help include:

- Preterm babies who have been given dummies for comfort over a long period of time, particularly if they refuse the breast.
- Preterm babies who have been given bottles before they are established at the breast. These babies may also initially refuse to breastfeed.
- Term babies who have been given bottles or dummies, and who refuse to breastfeed because they may have developed a preference for the stimulation provided by a teat.

2.2   How long should a feed last?

Clocks have no place in timing feeds for term healthy babies. If a baby is in the correct position and suckling properly, the feed should last until the baby is satisfied and comes off the breast himself. No two babies will feed for the same length of time. A term baby should have as long as he wants on the first breast and should then be offered the other breast, which may or may not be taken. At each feed, the baby should be given alternate breasts so that each breast is equally stimulated. Some mothers find it helps them to remember which breast to start the feed from if they attach a safety pin or brooch on the appropriate side of their clothing.

In the case of preterm babies, and particularly those of 35 weeks or less and sick babies, it is equally important not to restrict the time they spend suckling at the breast. It is quite satisfactory not to offer the other breast if the baby is satisfied. As with the term healthy baby, alternate breasts should be offered to the baby at each feed (although it may, in this case, be necessary to express the milk from the other side if the baby is not yet taking all the milk he requires from the breast).

Whilst no time limit should be placed on a breastfeed, there are situations, particularly with babies less than 34 or 35 weeks, or who have cardiac or respiratory problems, where feeds are obviously taking too long. One and a half hours, for example, would not be normal for the majority of babies.

Poor or static weight gain is often associated with prolonged feeding times and a further indication that a problem exists.

If the breastfeeds are taking a very long time, there are a number of possible reasons:

- Bad positioning and attachment of the baby at the breast.
- A poor maternal milk supply, owing to a lack of effective stimulation.
- The baby has an immature or weak pattern of sucking, and is not able to drain the lactiferous sinuses or breast effectively.
- The baby has a clinical condition, making him sleepy or weak.

2.2.1 Remedies to use when feeding times are prolonged

- Ensure the baby is in an appropriate position for feeding according to his size and gestation. Check the baby is attached to the breast and **not** sucking only on the nipple. Teach the mother to support/cup her baby's head with one hand so that when he opens his mouth widely she can use her other hand to guide her nipple and areola into his mouth, taking her hand away once attachment is achieved.

- If the baby has a weak, immature or uncoordinated suckling action, appropriate sucking practice may help – ideally this should be at the breast. A clean index or little finger may help you diagnose whether there is any uncoordinated tongue movement. Gently agitate the area between the baby's hard and soft palate with the pad of the finger. This should stimulate a sucking response. The finger should not be so far back in the baby's mouth that he gags. The tongue should move in a rhythmic way from the front to the back. Allow the baby to suck on your knuckle if possible for about half a minute before a feed.

- Examine the mother's present routine, particularly if she has recently gone home from hospital. She may be spending a lot of time trying to get back into a 'normal routine' thus reducing the regularity or length of expression or breastfeeding sessions. She may not be eating or drinking regularly if she has to visit her baby in a neonatal unit or has other children to care for. She may feel she has to do all the things she did before her baby also needed her, and may need help and support to recognize that her priorities are now likely to be different – and that one of her important priorities is to care for **herself**. She also needs to accept that life is unlikely to return to how it was before her baby was born.

- A mother of a baby with low energy reserves may find it beneficial to learn how to hand express, so that she can use 'direct expression' to start a breastfeed. If the mother has a good milk supply she should express a small quantity of milk prior to feeding, so that her baby obtains the fat-rich hind-milk more quickly. The milk already expressed may be given to the baby in a cup after the breastfeed, as this will require little energy expenditure. This regime aims at increasing the baby's weight without the baby becoming too tired to feed orally.

- A jaundiced baby may be too sleepy to feed, in which case it will be counterproductive to try to wake him. It may be better to wait until he wakes naturally or, if there is any concern that the baby's condition will worsen as a result, to give him a feed by gastric tube.

2.3   How often should a baby feed?

Babies born at term who are healthy and for whom there is no medical contraindication should feed whenever they are hungry or thirsty, that is, 'on demand'. No time intervals should be imposed. This may mean that some babies sleep for quite long periods between breastfeeds in the first few days after birth. Thereafter, the frequency of feeding between individual babies may vary enormously. Some babies may feed as often as 10–12 times in 24 hours, while others may only feed 5–6 times. Both are normal. In a neonatal or paediatric unit feeding regimens are rarely 'normal'; they exist to enable a set quantity of fluid to be given to a baby over a 24 hour period – left alone a baby may have other ideas of how often he wishes to feed. Very occasionally the two may be the same!

There is evidence to suggest that babies who are unrestricted in frequency of feeds gain weight more rapidly.[2] On a neonatal unit a 3 or 4 hourly feeding schedule may be considered necessary for some breastfed babies because of an existing clinical condition, such as jaundice, although if a baby has to be woken, he will be less inclined to feed properly and take the full amounts. It is better to let the baby regulate himself as soon as possible.

If the baby is being tube fed overnight, it is important to make sure the feeds are given **regularly** i.e. 3 hourly, so that more flexibility of timing feeds is possible during the day when the mother is available to feed. Daily or alternate day weighing is an appropriate way of assessing the baby's progress and detecting any feeding problems.

Many babies do eventually establish a pattern of between 5 and 6 feeds in 24 hours, with more frequent feeds often required towards the evening. Night feeds are very important and mothers should not be encouraged to miss them whilst in hospital. Otherwise, once the mother and her baby return home, she may be totally unprepared for her baby's normal feeding pattern. Night feeds also help maintain her milk supply, particularly in the early days, by stimulating the production of prolactin.

During periods of rapid growth, which will occur in the first 2–3 months post-delivery, a baby may want extra feeds. This often coincides with the time that many mothers give up breastfeeding, because they mistakenly believe their milk supply is no longer sufficient for the baby, who has suddenly become rather irritable and appears unsatisfied with his usual feeding regime. This unsettled period lasts for 24–48 hours whilst the mother's milk supply adjusts to her baby's new needs. The routine then usually returns to the 'normal' feeding pattern for that baby.

Term babies who are having antibiotic therapy but who are otherwise well should be fed on 'demand'. For term babies who are unwell, but are waking and requiring feeds, 'demand' feeding is more suitable as they may require extra fluids and calories. A formal time schedule may interfere with this by restricting their fluid intake. Most jaundiced term babies will also be able to regulate their own feeding requirements.

2.3.1   The preterm baby

Babies of 36 weeks gestation or less, and who are exclusively breastfeeding or having tube/cup feeds overnight should be allowed to go 3–4 hours between feeds, as long as this is not medically contraindicated. Alternate daily weights are recommended for this group of babies if fed on demand.

Preterm babies may initially require continuous pump feeds, until they are able to tolerate bolus feeds at 1, 2 or 3 hourly intervals. Once they can tolerate 2 hourly bolus feeds it is a mistake to believe that they **will** all eventually tolerate 3 hourly feeds. While it is common for 3 hourly feeds to be introduced during the time the baby is on a neonatal unit, it is essential for a mother to be aware that, when the baby goes home, he may feed according to his own individual needs (and these may be more frequent feeds – 10 or more breastfeeds in 24 hours is not unusual). It is **not** a sign that the mother has an insufficient milk supply. As with babies born at term, a 3–4 hourly pattern often emerges **but not always**, and when it does not happen, it is for that particular baby, his own personal pattern of feeding.

2.4   Has the baby had sufficient?

A baby who settles well between feeds, has at least 4–6 wet nappies per day and is putting on weight is getting sufficient milk! It is usual for babies to lose some weight in the first week of life. By day 10–14, most healthy term babies will have regained their birthweight. This will not apply if a baby is very preterm or very poorly – it may then take longer for the baby to regain his birthweight. How much longer will depend on the individual circumstances of the baby.

During the first week to 10 days, whilst the mother is still experiencing the feeling of breast fullness prior to feeding, it is useful to encourage her to gently handle her breasts to get to know how they feel before and after a feed. This will give her the confidence to know her baby has had sufficient milk. She can be assured that, if her breasts are soft and comfortable following a feed, then her baby is getting sufficient milk – particularly if the points at the beginning of the first paragraph are taken into consideration.

2.5 The baby's need for oral stimulation

In utero babies have practice and experience of sucking and swallowing so that, when born at term, most are capable of breastfeeding within a very short time of birth.

For the preterm baby, depending upon his gestation at birth, this opportunity to 'prime' the structures involved in feeding is incomplete. However, many preterm babies show a desire for oral stimulation of some kind. It is particularly noticeable, for example, in some preterm babies that they open and close their mouths and protrude their tongue during intermittent gastric tube feeds. This may be due to subtle temperature changes experienced by the baby during the feed.

Some preterm babies who are ventilated for any length of time may have considerable oral stimulation from the endotracheal tube, consequently some are able to suckle quite well after extubation (even a baby as young as 28 weeks post-conception age who is held close to the mother's breast after extubation may lick any milk expressed on to the nipple and some may attempt to suckle). This appears to be a 'temporary' skill, however, which disappears quite quickly, only to reappear when the baby is more mature and developmentality more able to co-ordinate his skills safely.

The question is what kind of oral stimulation should be given to a baby who is preterm, sick or has an oral defect? For the preterm baby there is a need to provide some form of developmentally appropriate stimulation, which at the same time provides comfort to the baby. For the sick baby who is term, the need for comfort may be very acute, and for the baby with an oral defect or a neurological condition it may be important to provide stimulation to the palate and tongue to encourage correct feeding movements. The kind of oral stimulation a baby receives, particularly if he is in a neonatal or paediatric unit, may be quite extensive. It may range from being very unpleasant, though necessary or even life saving – for example, oral intubation, oral suctioning, the making and fitting of a dental plate (or obdurator), the passing of oral gastric feeding tubes, perhaps even mouth care – to being a positive and pleasurable stimulation, such as licking milk from the nipple or suckling at the breast. It may include sucking on a dummy, a bottle teat, a nipple shield, a finger or the baby's own fist, taking milk from a cup, or from the tube of a nursing supplementer.

What has to be considered for each individual baby is what kind of oral stimulation is absolutely necessary; what is preferable as far as the establishment of breastfeeding is concerned and what should be avoided if possible. A point of conflict in assessing the needs of a baby who is to breastfeed is how to provide oral stimulation which can comfort him if his mother is not present, or which can calm him when, for example, he exhibits signs of wanting something in his mouth at the time of being gastrically tube fed.

It is important to distinguish the baby's possible need for oral 'gratification', which may require some form of oral stimulation, and his need to be comforted. For a baby who is to be breastfed, both needs can be provided by the mother. Therefore, it is important for her to introduce her baby to the breast as early as possible. A baby will derive a lot of comfort from suckling as well as satisfying his oral and nutritive needs. Whether the baby is sick or preterm, comfort can be provided in a number of ways – even when the mother is not present. Sometimes it is tempting to give a baby a dummy when what the baby really wants is to be held and spoken to or caressed. A mother or a health professional can carry a baby in a sling. Sometimes all that is required is a tape recording of his parents' voices or gentle music or sounds, or even a breast pad or piece of clothing with his mother's familiar breast scent.

If the baby is obviously looking for some sort of oral stimulation and his mother is not present it may be appropriate to give him a cup-feed (rather than a gastric tube feed and a dummy). A cup-feed will stimulate his tongue, lingual lipases, and his oral and nasal sensory receptors without expecting him to have anything in his mouth which he may find difficult to control, particularly if he is still very immature (30–32 weeks gestation, for example). A cup-feed may be especially appropriate for a baby with an oral defect or a neurological condition, who needs to strengthen his oral musculature and encourage a rhythmic tongue movement.

The tongue is a very important sensory organ capable of providing pleasurable experiences. It is therefore important to use it to help a baby who has been subjected to any of the unpleasant oral stimuli previously mentioned. Cup-feeding makes use of the tongue: it encourages its movement in order to obtain the milk from the cup. All that is in the mouth is milk (preferably the mother's breastmilk). Furthermore, cup-feeding provides a 'self-regulated' oral experience. If the baby is stimulated he takes milk, if he is not, he takes none. It is useful to provide a baby with an oral feeding experience which will not interfere with breastfeeding, but at the same time will satisfy his need for oral stimulation and require the person giving the feed to talk to and to hold the baby.

When a baby breastfeeds a similar 'self-regulation' process occurs, for it is the baby who decides on the pace of the feed, when to begin and when to finish suckling. For a preterm baby who still has to learn to breastfeed, the best oral stimulation is provided at his mother's breast. Skin-to-skin contact is very beneficial for it gives the baby ready access to the breast. The mother can express a little milk on to her nipples, or express directly into her baby's mouth and she can help him attach to the breast. If he is sick, with very little energy, or still very young (32–35 weeks gestation) he may be content simply to hold the breast tissue in his mouth. Suckling may not occur until he is ready, which may not be for several days or even weeks. The baby will decide when he is ready for another kind of oral stimulation and often this will be dictated by his own individual developmental 'clock'. The significance of this is not to force an immature baby to do anything he is not yet ready to do. Orally, this means avoiding the use of bottles until a baby is able to cope with them. As the skill of cup-feeding appears to precede efficient breastfeeding, and breastfeeding appears to be possible before bottle-feeding it may be prudent to avoid bottles altogether or at least until the baby and his mother have breastfeeding well established.

Oral stimulation can enhance or detract from the establishment of breastfeeding.[4,5] Dummies are often used in neonatal and paediatric units, but they are not pliable like the breast. They are static in the mouth and do not encourage the same movements of the tongue, lips or oral muscles as required in suckling. This is also true of the bottle teat, nipple shield and a finger. Nevertheless, there may be times when any one of these forms of oral stimulation is used (the bottle and dummy preferably with the permission of the parents). Where possible their use should be minimized so that the predominant oral stimulation experienced by a baby is at his mother's breast.

References

1   WHO/UNICEF (1993) *Breastfeeding Counselling: A Training Course.* Secretariat, Division of Diarrhoeal and Acute Respiratory Disease Control, Session 3 pp. 39–54. WHO, Geneva, Switzerland.
2   Illingworth RS and Stone DG (1952) Self-demand feeding in a Maternity Unit. *Lancet* **1**: 683–687.
3   Bernbaum JC, Pereira GR, Watkins JB and Peckham GJ (1983) Non-nutritive sucking during gavage feeding enhances growth and maturation in preterm babies. *Pediatrics* **71**: 41–45.
4   Victora CG, Tomasi E, Olinto MTA and Barros FC (1993) Use of pacifiers and breastfeeding duration. *Lancet* **341**: 401–406.
5   Righard L and Alade MO (1992) Sucking technique and its effect on success of breastfeeding. *Birth* **19**: 185–189.

3 The expression of breastmilk

3.1 Hand expression

The expression of breastmilk by hand is a skill which **all** mothers who are going to breastfeed should have the opportunity of acquiring.

The reasons for teaching a mother to hand express are:

- It ensures a mother is able to handle her breasts correctly. This will initially help her to know how her breasts feel before and after a feed – giving her confidence about how much milk her baby has taken at a breastfeed.
- To give a mother confidence that her body is working normally. She may feel that her body has failed her, if she has given birth to a preterm or sick baby.
- To give a mother control over her own body and its milk production.
- To enable a mother to express sufficient milk for a feed if her baby cannot be breastfed, either immediately after birth or on a later occasion, for example, if the mother returns to work, or the mother or baby become ill.
- To enable a mother to express milk straight into her baby's mouth. This is useful when the baby is preterm and just beginning to learn to feed because it stimulates his digestive juices (including the lingual lipases), and encourages the movement of his tongue and jaw muscles.
- It may help a baby to attach at the breast if a little milk is expressed on to the mother's nipple. This is particularly helpful for the preterm baby when he is learning to feed, or for a baby who tires quickly. It may also be useful for babies with Down's syndrome, and babies with a cleft lip and/or palate abnormalities.
- To enable the expression of some fore-milk if the mother

has an abundant milk supply and the baby is unable to obtain the fat-rich hind-milk because he has low energy reserves and cannot yet complete a feed.

- To express any lobes of the breast which become blocked. It is, therefore one of the 'first aid' measures in preventing mastitis. (It may be used in conjunction with massage, see Section 3.6 of this chapter.)
- To express a little milk prior to a feed to soften the mother's nipples, if they have become flattened due to engorgement or breast fullness. This will help a baby to attach to the breast correctly.
- Some mothers may find a small amount of hind-milk gently smoothed over the nipple area after a feed or expression helps prevent the delicate skin from becoming too dry.
- Some mothers find hand expression more relaxing and more acceptable than using a mechanical pump.
- Hand-expressed milk **may** result in milk with a higher sodium content and concentration than pump-expressed milk.[1] This may be advantageous to preterm babies of less than 30 weeks gestation, who may have excessive sodium loss, owing to an immature renal function.[2]

3.1.1   When and how often to hand express

If a baby is unable to be breastfed after birth, for whatever reason, expression of milk is usually necessary, by hand or pump. This should be commenced on the day of birth (if possible), in the same way as breastfeeding. The **colostrum** produced in these first days is very important for all babies, and particularly for those born preterm or who are sick.

Therefore, when breastfeeding cannot begin within a few hours of birth, milk should be expressed:

- As soon after birth as possible.
- At least 6–8 times in a 24 hour period, sometimes more.
- During the night.

No time limits should be set because the length of expression will vary with each mother.

Practically, it is much easier to teach a mother the principles of hand expression when her breasts are soft. If she does not begin expression until day 3 or 4, she is less likely to learn the skill easily, because it may be more uncomfortable and even painful to learn when there is venous engorgement and her breasts are full of milk.

There is good evidence[3] to suggest that the earlier a mother begins to express, the more successful she will be at maintaining lactation over long periods of time. Another reason for teaching hand expression very early in the post-natal period is to ensure the mother knows what to do **before** any problems arise. If a situation then occurs which requires expression, she is already familiar with the principles of expressing by hand, and does not have to learn how to do it at a time when she is either tense, uncomfortable or in pain. Therefore, where the mother may be discharged from hospital care within 24 hours of delivering her baby, she is best taught in this very early period.

3.1.2 How to hand express

There are several different ways to hand express. A mother needs to practise and perfect her own technique, although first of all she has to learn the 'principles' underlying the practice, which are the same for **all** mothers. The techniques are 'refinements', which vary according to individual preference, and which work for some mothers and not for others.

It is important that the mother achieves success at hand expression from the beginning, because it teaches her many more skills than simply removing milk from the breast. For example, if hand expression is taught **before** the baby is able to feed from the breast, then the mother is able to hold her breast in an appropriate way to help the baby become attached when he is ready.

Before a mother hand expresses she should:

- Wash her hands thoroughly. There is no need for her to wash her breasts more than once a day.
- Have a prepared sterile container for her milk. It is preferable to use a bottle or cup which can then be stored without having to transfer the milk into another container. Some mothers may find a wide-necked container useful while still perfecting their technique.

The following suggestions may help a mother to be well prepared and successful at the time of expression.

- Have a damp clean cloth and paper tissues nearby, for her hands, accidental splashes of milk or spillage.
- Have a drink prepared.
- If parted from her baby have a photograph of him nearby.
- Be as relaxed as possible, listen to music or something which makes her laugh, sit in a really comfortable chair, have low lighting when expressing in the evening!
- Express in a warm room.
- Express while in a warm bath!

The principles of hand expression (Fig. 3.1):

1. Place the fingers of one hand under the breast. The little finger can be placed against the chest wall, and the other fingers spread evenly under the breast towards the nipple, supporting the breast.
2. Place the thumb on the top of the breast just behind the areola, opposite the first finger.

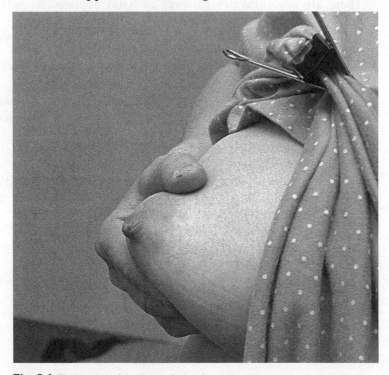

Fig. 3.1 *The position of the fingers for hand expression.*

3. Gently agitate/palpate the first finger and thumb, feeling the nature of the underlying tissue. Try to locate the small fibrous thickenings or grape-like structures. These are usually situated beneath, or at the margins of, the areola and behind the nipple. These are the lactiferous sinuses. Pressure should be applied just behind these sinuses or, if they cannot be located, then just behind the areola.

4. To remove the milk from the sinuses, compress and release the breast tissue with the thumb and fingers. This action should be repeated regularly. The speed, pressure and rhythm of this will vary according to each mother.

5. To express sufficient milk for a feed, the thumb and forefinger need to move around the outside edge of the sinuses or areola to ensure all the lactiferous sinuses are drained (Fig. 3.2).

6. Movement on the skin should be avoided, this is an extremely sensitive part of the body and can be easily damaged by rough handling.

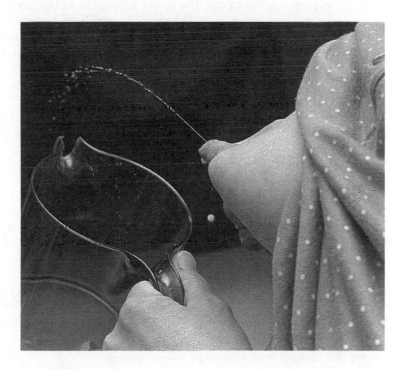

Fig. 3.2 *The expression of milk.*

Possible additions to and variations of the principles of hand expression

- Gently press inwards towards the chest wall when using the compress–release movement.
- Gentle shaking of the breasts,[4] when leaning over may help to enhance the milk flow.
- Using both hands on either side of the breast, rather than only one hand as described above (see Fig. 3.3).
- Place one hand flat on the top of the breast and the other hand flat under the breast. Without moving the hands, apply simultaneous compress and release movements.
- Gently roll the thumb or forefinger from side to side towards the nipple. At the same time compress and release, compress and release.
- Express from both breasts at the same time into a wide-necked container or two separate containers, one under each breast. Lean forward, with the breasts hanging loosely over the container (see Fig. 3.4). This will help in expressing milk from the lower lobes. The container can be secured between the mother's knees. Both breasts can be expressed simultaneously with frequent pauses to let the lactiferous sinuses fill with milk, or they can be expressed alternately.

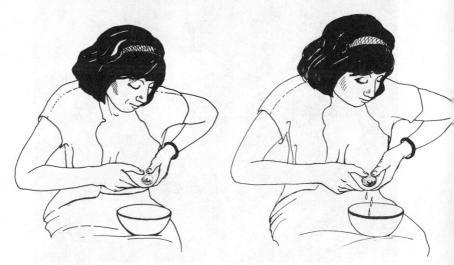

Fig. 3.3 *Expression of the breast using a two-hand technique.*

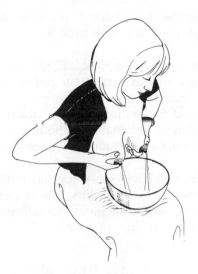

Fig. 3.4 *A position for hand expression of both breasts.*

What to expect at an individual expression session

1. With the first few compress–release movements of an expression it is possible that no milk will be immediately visible (particularly in the initial period after birth when colostrum is present).
2. As the movements continue, small amounts of milk will begin to appear at different places on the tip of the nipple.
3. With further compress–release movements, the milk is likely to spurt from the nipple from several different ducts.
4. Gradually the spurts will become less forceful, until there are only drips of milk. Then move the thumb and forefinger around to drain other sinuses.
5. Repeat the procedure with the other breast. Alternate between the breasts when the milk flow slows (this occurs approximately every 2–4 minutes).

- Milk volume will be increased by alternating the expression between the breasts in the way described above.

- Gentle simultaneous hand massage at the time of expression may help with milk flow.

In the first few days of expression, when colostrum is present, it may just drip into a container and not spurt, because it is thicker than mature milk. In a few mothers, the milk does not spurt. Instead the milk flow is a steady and consistent stream. This is quite acceptable, although it is important to check that the mother's technique is appropriate for efficient expression.

Some mothers will have colostrum and milk dripping from the nipple before expression begins. This is completely normal and these mothers should be given the information beginning at (3) of the above sequence of events.

3.1.3   How to teach a mother to hand express

There are a number of ways to teach a mother the skill of hand expression:

1. She can be verbally instructed in the principles, by going very carefully through each stage.
2. She can be given written instructions.
3. She can be shown what to do:

    - Using a model breast.
    - By the person teaching, illustrating the movements using her own body.
    - The mother can be shown using her own breast.

Using the mother's own breast ensures that she sees how simple the skill of hand expression is, and knows how it feels for herself. The mother only needs to be touched on this one occasion. Once she has mastered hand expression and how to position her fingers, the mother is able, with minimal instruction, to attach her baby herself, without the need for the baby to be attached for her.

A combination of all three methods is likely to be the most successful. However, whichever method is chosen, it is still important to observe the mother expressing, to be sure she has a safe technique. It is useful for the mother to also have written instructions for reference.

Practical instruction

If you and the mother decide that the demonstration will be
carried out on the mother's breast, show her with **your hand**
on **her breast** in the exact position she will need to hold **her
hand**. This means standing either slightly behind the mother
or to her side (see Fig. 3.5). Once you have expressed milk on
to her nipple, ask the mother to cover your hand with hers,
and then withdraw your hand. The mother's hand should now
be in exactly the same position on her breast as your hand was.
She can then continue to express from this breast, before initiat-
ing the milk flow from the other breast. Once this process has
been completed, the mother can be told of the various 'refinements' she can add to the basic principles, which she can then
practice in her own time.

Practice will perfect the mother's technique of hand
expression. It may not work perfectly the first time she does it.

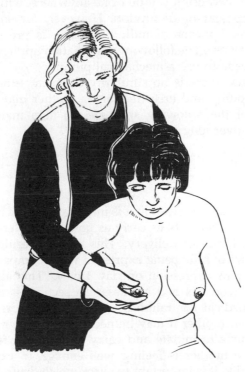

Fig. 3.5 *Where to stand when teaching a mother to hand express.*

However, it is worth investing time in teaching the 'principles' to the mother and in her acquiring the skill. She will certainly benefit from the help she is given.

In circumstances where the mother cannot or does not want to express her milk by pump, and she has difficulties with hand expression, her partner can be taught the skill and help the mother to express her milk.

3.2 When and how to use a mechanical pump

Expression of breastmilk may be necessary in a number of situations, some of which require the mother to express for several weeks, for example, if she has a baby born at less than 27 weeks gestation. For many mothers, a mechanical pump helps them to express breastmilk in sufficient volumes, over the many weeks until their babies are able to suckle effectively from the breast. Hand expression gives the mother a degree of social freedom because it can be done anywhere, with the minimum of equipment or disruption. However, for some mothers, a mechanical means of milk expression is preferable for most everyday use. The following information applies to **any** mother who needs to use a mechanical pump.

Because there is no similarity between using a mechanical breast pump and breastfeeding, a mother may need to adopt some of the following strategies to help maintain her milk supply over long periods of time.

3.2.1 When to pump

As with hand expression, it is important for the mother to begin expressing her milk as early as possible, preferably within the first 24 hours of delivery. This usually results in improved quantities of milk being expressed when compared to a mother who begins expression on day 3 or 4.[3] This also applies to a mother who has had a Caesarean section – unless there are good medical contraindications to early expression. For this particular mother it may be necessary for the midwife or neonatal nurse to initiate and carry out the first few expressions until the mother is feeling well enough to express her own breastmilk. It is important to check which drugs the mother has been given and whether they may adversely affect the breastmilk. Even if they do, the expression should still be commenced early to stimulate the milk supply – but the milk may need to be **discarded**.

The colostrum[5,6] obtained in the first few days should be given to the baby immediately, or at the earliest opportunity after expression, preferably as a bolus feed, for it has many medicinal qualities.[7]

How often?

To ensure an adequate milk supply over any length of time, expression should be maintained 2–3 hourly for a minimum of six times in 24 hours.[3] Sometimes more frequent expression may be necessary if the milk supply begins to diminish.

Expression should be started soon after the mother gets up in the morning and, to ensure the gap is not too long overnight, it should be one of the last things she does before going to bed. The other expressions should be spaced equally throughout the day. Ideally the mother should express in the night as well.[8] While she is in hospital it is **the mother** who should decide if she wishes to be woken to express breastmilk or to feed her baby, not the staff. It is important that the mother does not go for longer than 6–7 hours overnight without expressing because she may become uncomfortably full by the morning, particularly in the early post-natal period. If this occurs regularly, her milk production may be inhibited which will gradually result in a decrease in milk volume.

How long?

Length of expression will vary between each mother but will commonly take between 10 and 20 minutes for each breast. On the first day a few minutes only on each side may be all the mother can tolerate. A time limit should not be specified and she should be advised to express her milk until the flow ceases. The expression of both breasts should not normally take longer than 1 hour. If this is happening, check the technique the mother is using.

The amount of milk produced

The volume of milk produced at each expression will vary throughout the day. The greatest volume being obtained in the morning, with lesser amounts obtained as the day proceeds. The volume may also vary according to the emotional state of the mother. In a neonatal or paediatric unit, for example, her baby's clinical condition may be unstable, causing the mother to be very stressed at times. Few mothers are aware of the normal differences in the diurnal milk flow and fewer still are aware that any emotional upset may temporarily reduce their milk flow (an effect frequently observed on neonatal units). It is important the mother is aware, so that she does not worry unnecessarily about her ability to lactate.

Colostrum appears to be produced in very small volumes, often no more than 5–20 ml per expression. For the needs of most term babies this is quite sufficient in the first few days after delivery and additional fluids are not normally required. This will apply, for example, if a baby is receiving antibiotics prophylactically, but is otherwise well – as in the case of a term baby whose mother had premature rupture of membranes (PROM).

A mother expressing her breastmilk may notice:

- The milk flow increases substantially over the first few days after birth, with the daily variation in milk volume obtained at each expression becoming more obvious.
- The milk supply may begin to diminish at around 10–14 days, particularly if she has been staying in hospital, near her baby from birth. This period often coincides with the mother going home and having many other pressures to cope with.

As long as the mother continues to receive constant support and reassurance, she should be able to maintain her supply.

3.2.2 How to pump

Once the basic method of using an electric or hand pump is explained to a mother, there are several tips that may help her maintain her supply and make expression more comfortable:

- Alternating the pumping of each breast every 4–5 minutes is shown to encourage the flow.
- The position of the cup at the breast, when expressing,

should be slightly changed at regular intervals to stimulate different lobes.

- Expression in a warm room will be beneficial. The mother may find placing a warm cloth over the breast may also help.
- Using a 'flexi-shield' (see Fig. 3.6). For some mothers this device provides a more comfortable means of expression than using the glass or plastic funnel on its own. The shield fits on to the rim of the funnel, and allows the mother to use the highest setting on the breast pump, which provides a more effective rhythm of expression.
- Expressing from one breast whilst feeding from the other may help a mother who has a diminished milk supply.
- 'Double pumping' allows expression to be completed more quickly (Fig. 3.7), it may be beneficial to have $\frac{1}{2}$ to 1 minute pauses during the session at 3–4 minute intervals, so that milk can drain into the lactiferous sinuses (this occurs where a pump does not have a pause mechanism built into it). 'Double pumping' is reported to encourage an increased milk supply and high prolactin levels when compared to other methods of expression.[9]

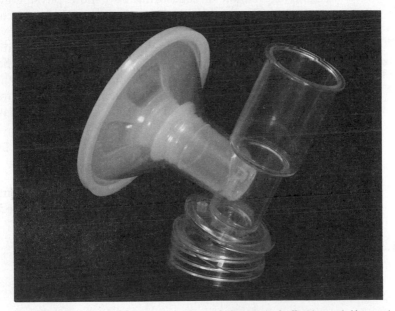

Fig. 3.6 *The flexi-shield. (Photo courtesy of the North Staffs Neonatal Unit and Egnell-Ameda.)*

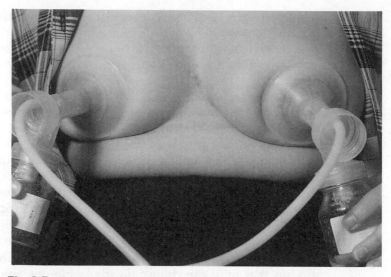

Fig. 3.7 *Expression using a pump with an attachment for 'double-pumping'. (Photo courtesy of the North Staffs Neonatal Unit and Egnell-Ameda.)*

(Mothers who hand express may also express from both breasts at the same time.)
- Hand expression of breastmilk is a more physiological technique than mechanical expression, and there is evidence to suggest that it results in higher prolactin levels than ordinary mechanical expression.[8,10] A combination of methods may be a useful compromise, with mechanical pumping performed for the first 5–10 minutes, and then expression by hand until there is no further milk flow. Any combination can be used, as long as it is satisfactory to the mother.
- Breast massage will help encourage milk flow if performed prior to expression.

Whichever method of breast expression the mother finds most comfortable, successful and acceptable should be used.

3.3   Storage of expressed breastmilk and its sequence of use

3.3.1   Containers and storage

1. A sterile container should be used for milk collection and storage.

2. The bottle should not be filled right to the top. At least 2.5 cm should be left at the top because, if the milk is to be frozen, it will expand.
3. Milk can be expressed into a separate container at each session. It can also be added to already frozen milk, as long as it is then put straight back into the freezer and the frozen milk is not allowed to defrost. It is suggested that the milk should be cooled before adding it to the frozen milk, so that the top layer does not thaw.
4. Each bottle should be labelled with the mother's name, date and time of expression.
5. Raw breastmilk (i.e. milk that has not been pasteurized) can be stored for between 24 and 48 hours in the refrigerator at 4°C, if it is to be used within this period of time.[12]
6. Freshly expressed breastmilk can be left at room temperature for 6-8 hours[13] although if it is not going to be used straightaway it should be refrigerated as soon as possible.
7. If it is not to be used within 24 hours, raw breastmilk should be stored in the freezer. It can be stored for 3 months at −20°C, after which time it should be discarded.

The effect of the container on milk composition

The containers used to store breastmilk may be made of glass, plastic or stainless steel. Several studies have reported that the type of container can affect the milk composition, in some cases certain constituents of the milk stick to the sides of the containers, for example lipids (fats) have been observed to stick to plastic storage bags.[14] Concern has also been expressed about the repeated cleaning of containers made of polypropylene, which can increase the risk of bacterial contamination[15] from scratches to the inside of the container.

Glass containers are recommended for storing expressed breastmilk. They do not appear to adversely affect the milk constituents and, although cells have been observed to stick to the sides of glass, they have also been observed to detach from the sides after 24 hours of storage.[16] Glass containers can be easily cleaned thus reducing the risk of contamination.

3.3.2   Defrosting breastmilk

1. Defrosting raw breastmilk is best achieved by putting the bottle of frozen milk into the refrigerator.[16]

2. When removed from the freezer, it should be labelled with the date and time. It should be used within 24 hours.
3. Frozen milk can also be defrosted by putting the bottle in running warm water.[16]
4. Defrosting breastmilk in a microwave is not recommended, as this may heat the milk unevenly with a potential risk of burning the baby's mouth and throat. Microwaving also destroys 30% of the protective immunoproteins.[16]

Do not refreeze milk once it is defrosted!

3.3.3   Sequence of breastmilk use

1. Use all colostrum.
2. Use the first 14 days of milk in order (there is still colostrum in this milk).
3. After this, use milk as it is produced, i.e. use fresh milk if possible or use the milk produced on the same day.
4. Where a mother produces more milk than her baby requires, use the milk in order of expression, for that day, and freeze the remainder, i.e. use the milk she produces in the morning before the milk produced in the afternoon or evening. The highest fat levels in human milk are generally found in milk expressed in the morning and early afternoon,[17] therefore this milk should be given to the baby.

Fewer bacteria are found in hand expressed milk than in mechanically expressed milk,[18] which reflects possible contamination from the equipment. This emphasizes the importance of ensuring that any breast-pump equipment used is properly cleaned and sterilized.

3.4   Prolonged expression of breastmilk

Any mother who has to express her milk for longer than 3 days will need some of the following information, in addition to information contained earlier in this chapter on expression. The information contained at the end of this section is particularly important for any mother who has to express her breastmilk over a period of weeks, rather than days.

Prolonged expression of milk may be necessary if a mother wishes to provide her own breastmilk for a preterm, sick or bottlefed baby. A number of potential problems can occur, depending upon the length of time over which the mother has to maintain her lactation. Her success depends upon a level of commitment, which is sometimes difficult to sustain, together with the support of her family, hospital staff and anyone else involved in her care.

3.4.1 Suggestions for reducing long-term problems

The following suggestions are aimed at reducing any long-term problems, which can arise from the prolonged expression of breastmilk:

- Advise the mother to express when she is in the unit with her baby, or in an atmosphere in which she can relax, listening to music, or with a photograph of her baby beside her.
- If or when the mother's milk does begin to diminish, reassure her that this is not a permanent state and urge her to continue expressing. Increasing the number of sessions of expression may help to increase her milk supply.
- Whilst it cannot be emphasized enough how important regular expressing is, it is necessary to recognize that the mother needs to have the occasional break. She can quite safely miss an expression as long as it is only an occasional break. Indeed, it is important she does take a break. If she is to be able to go out and still maintain regular expression, she may find the electric pump useful at home, and hand expression useful when she is out.
- Hand expression is a useful and tactile method of expressing and should be used whenever possible. If the mother uses an electric pump, encourage her to hand express **after** she thinks that she has finished on the pump. She will almost certainly see that she still has milk and, if she can become proficient in expressing this, it is nutritionally very important for her baby.
- It is worth a mother experimenting with different methods of expressing to find the most appropriate method for her. It may be that the method she is using is not the best for her and this may be causing or appearing to cause a diminished milk supply.
- Suggest to the mother that she keeps a record of the

amounts that she expresses. She may well be encouraged to see that she has more milk than she thinks she has! If her milk supply has diminished, she may see a positive result from the advice given to her.

- Whenever possible, it is worth reminding the mother that, as each day passes, her baby is either becoming more mature, growing and getting stronger, or, if he is recovering from an illness, getting better. This brings breastfeeding closer and the prospect of the baby being able to stimulate his mother's milk supply on his own.
- Massage of the breasts prior to pumping for 3–5 minutes will stimulate the blood supply and may therefore encourage the milk supply.
- Very gentle massage of the nipple for $\frac{1}{2}$ minute may stimulate the release of prolactin and oxytocin, and, therefore, helps with the milk production and 'let-down' reflex. The nipple can either be rolled gently between the thumb and forefinger (see Fig. 3.8), or the palm of the hand can be gently moved back and forth over the tip of the nipple.
- Encourage the mother's partner or a friend to massage her back. It is suggested that this may help stimulate the release of oxytocin and the 'let-down' reflex.[19]

Back massage

There are several methods of back massage. The following three methods are easy to do and can involve a partner. They are also reported to be very pleasant for the mother. It may be

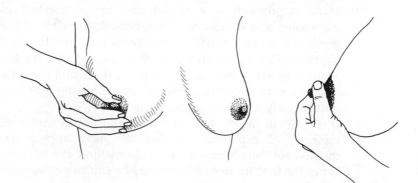

Fig. 3.8 *Nipple stimulation using the thumb and forefinger.*

advisable for a mother to have a container nearby or placed on her lap as milk will sometimes begin to flow spontaneously during back massage.

Method 1   (Fig. 3.9)

1. The mother should sit down, fold her arms in front of her on a table and rest her head on her arms. Her back should be exposed.
2. The person conducting the massage places the knuckles of both hands at the top of the mother's back, between her shoulder blades, and on either side of the spine.
3. The knuckles should be facing each other.
4. Using fairly brisk movements, move the knuckles in opposite directions, i.e. with one knuckle beginning at the top of the back and massaging to the bottom of the shoulder blades and the other knuckle beginning at the

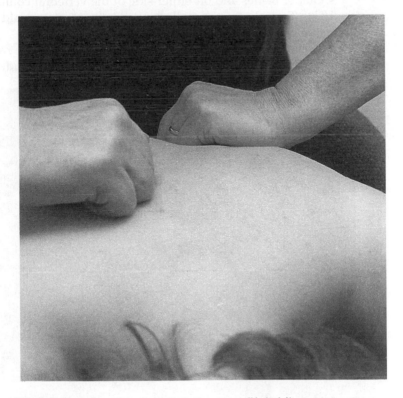

Fig. 3.9 *The position of the hands for back massage (Method 1).*

bottom of theshoulder blades and massaging to the top of the back.
5. Continue for about 3–4 minutes, or for however long is acceptable to the mother!

Although it is possible to do this massage over clothing, friction can make the skin on the knuckles very raw. It is better to use a little body oil directly on the skin of the back. If aromatherapy or homeopathic products are preferred, it is advisable to consult a qualified practitioner.

Method 2   (Fig. 3.10)

1. The mother should sit down, fold her arms in front of her on a table and rest her head on her arms.
2. The person conducting the massage uses the thumbs, beginning at the top of the mother's back, between her shoulder blades and on either side of the vertebral column.
3. Using firm pressure, small circular movements should be made with the thumbs.
4. Both sides of the spine are massaged at the same time, from the top of the back to the bottom of the shoulder blades.

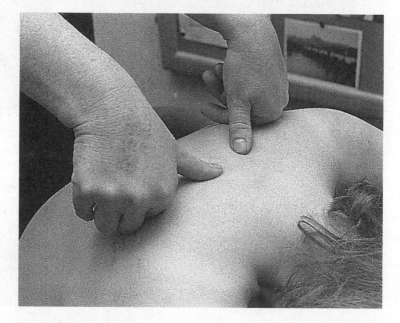

Fig. 3.10 *The position of the hands for back massage (Method 2).*

5.   Continue for about 3–4 minutes.

Method 3

This is a very simple massage.

1.   Place one hand flat on the top of the back, in the same position as for method 1.
2.   Place the other hand flat on the back approximately two-thirds of the way down the back.
3.   Using firm, smooth strokes, slide the hand at the top of the back down to the other hand.
4.   Swap hands and begin again. Continue in this way for a few minutes.

3.4.2   How to stop using a pump

A mother who is about to stop expressing her milk by mechanical pump should wean off the pump gradually, rather than very suddenly. This is particularly important where she has consistently produced more milk than her baby needs. This gives the breasts time to respond naturally to her baby's requirements. This process appears to take a few days, if the mother has been using a pump for several weeks.

When a mother suddenly stops using a mechanical pump, the milk may not be removed in sufficient quantities by her baby. This can lead to engorgement and, if it occurs continually, to mastitis.

Weaning off the pump

This is particularly important for any mother who:

- Has been expressing by mechanical pump for 2 weeks or more.
- Expresses more milk than her baby needs.

1.   Weaning off the pump should take place over a 4–5 day period, **not** abruptly.
2.   If possible the process should be completed whilst the baby is still in a hospital unit, therefore, it needs to be commenced approximately 5–6 days prior to the baby's discharge.

3. The milk expressed can be given by cup if required or stored.
4. The amount of milk to be expressed depends upon the mother's milk supply.
5. Write down the regime to be used by the mother.
6. Expression should be completed **before** breastfeeding takes place.

A sample regime   The volumes used in this sample regime are intended as examples only. How much breastmilk an individual mother expresses prior to each breastfeeding session will depend upon how much milk she was expressing before the establishment of breastfeeding began.

Day 1:
- Express 20–30 ml of breastmilk in total from both breasts, i.e. 10–15 ml from each breast in the morning, before breastfeeding.
- Express 15–25 ml of breastmilk in total, in the afternoon, before breastfeeding.
- Express 10–20 ml of breastmilk in total, in the evening, before breastfeeding.

It is important to use hand expression or a hand pump to express these amounts. **Do not** use an electric pump as this will usually maintain or increase production, not reduce it.

Day 2–5:
- Express as for day 1, but reduce the amounts expressed by:
- 5 ml of breastmilk in the morning
- 2–3 ml of breastmilk in the afternoon and evening.

Day 6:
- Do not express any milk before feeding from the breast.

This regime can be repeated if a baby does not continue to gain weight steadily, or if his weight gain becomes static or falls slightly.

To repeat the regime, reduce the amount of breastmilk expressed in the sample regime by approximately 5 ml at each expression. For example:

Day 1:
- Express 15–20 ml of breastmilk in the morning rather than 20–30 ml.

- Express 10–20 ml of breastmilk in the afternoon.
- Express 5–15 ml of breastmilk in the evening.

Then likewise reduce the expressions of day 2–5 by a further 5 ml at each expression.

3.5 Types of pump

There are a range of pumps available to mothers for hospital use or for use at home. In hospitals the most common pumps are electrically operated. These pumps either use a single funnel connection to remove the milk from one breast at a time, or have two funnel connections so that the milk can be removed simultaneously from both breasts ('double pumping'). Hand-held pumps, which use batteries or are operated by hand movements, are of many different designs, although they all have a funnel connection at the breast. There is no one type of hand pump that is ideal for all mothers. It is, therefore, particularly valuable if, while still in hospital and before a mother is tempted to buy a hand pump, she is given the opportunity to use a variety of designs which are available on a unit, to see which pump is most suitable for her needs (they are expensive, especially if once purchased they do not work for her!).

Hand pumps and hand expression are useful if a mother returns to work, or to give the mother more social freedom.

3.6 Breast massage

Breast massage complements hand expression. There are several ways to massage – each equally successful. In a neonatal unit, it is important to teach a mother a method that will not damage the skin or underlying tissues. This is particularly important when massage may be used long term.

3.6.1 Why is it necessary?

- It encourages a good blood flow to the breast and may therefore encourage an efficient milk supply.[20]
- It effectively helps disperse engorged lobes and mastitis.
- It helps a mother to relax. If she is feeling tired, anxious and/or has a poor milk supply, 4–5 minutes of gentle massage before a feed or expression will help calm her, and focus her mind on her milk.

- If Method 1 is taught, it can be performed over clothing using only one hand. This can be useful if the mother has other small children who want to be cuddled or read to at the same time!
- It is easy for a partner to learn and do.
- It is easy to massage whilst feeding or expressing, to encourage the milk flow.
- There is some evidence to suggest that, if gentle nipple stimulation is also used with the massage, it may help improve a diminished milk supply (owing to increased prolactin release, particularly if performed prior to mechanical pumping or hand expression).[21] Sometimes the nipple stimulation alone will result in milk beginning to flow from the breast.

3.6.2   How to massage

There are no right or wrong ways to massage. Some methods may be more successful with some mothers than others, but it is important to be **gentle**, particularly if the technique favoured by a mother allows her to move her hands over her skin.

The first method is useful prior to a feed or expression, because it enables all lobes of the breast to be massaged, and can be performed using only one hand without the need to remove any clothing. Either hand can be used according to ease. In addition no damage from friction can occur.

The second method is very gentle, it is useful during expression or to help disperse a blocked lobe. This method is also performed using only one hand but is more effective when used directly on the skin.

Method I

1. Clench the fist, placing the thumb end at the top of the breast towards the chest wall. Hold the fist at right angles to the chest (Fig. 3.11(a)).
2. Using a rolling action, roll the fist down the breast towards the nipple, transferring the pressure as this is done. Never roll in the opposite direction, because this will interfere with efficient breast drainage (Fig. 3.11(b)).
3. When massaging lobes under the breast, place the little finger end of the fist at the chest wall and roll the fist

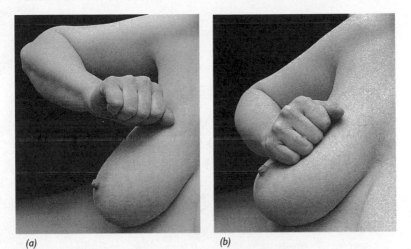

(a)   (b)

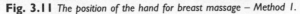

Fig. 3.11 *The position of the hand for breast massage – Method 1.*

upwards towards the nipple. If the breast is large or pendulous, an alternative way is to use a flat hand. Place the little finger next to the chest wall and gently roll the palm of the hand towards the nipple.
4. The pressure should be firm but gentle. If it is painful, **stop** and apply less pressure. It should be comfortable. It is very easy and effective.

Method 2[4]

1. The first two fingers of the hand are used for the opposite breast, so that the right hand massages the left breast and vice versa (Fig. 3.12).
2. Starting near the chest wall, lightly press the first two fingers gently into the breast tissue making small circular movements, without moving the fingers over the skin.
3. Gradually move the fingers towards the areola.
4. Using these movements, massage all around the breast.
5. Gently vibrating the fingers during the massage may make it more effective.

Always show the mother first, using your hand either on her breast or on yours. Be gentle but firm!

Other methods of massage

These include:
- Placing a flat hand on the top of the breast, and the other

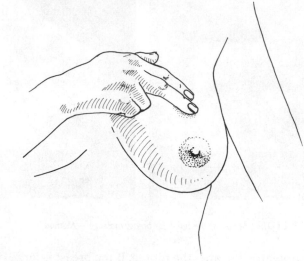

Fig. 3.12 *Massage of the breast – method 2.*

hand under the breast, and then either transferring pressure (as in Method 1), or gently moving the top hand over
the breast in sweeping movements towards the nipple
using the hand under the breast for support (see Fig. 3.13).
* Using the tips of all the fingers to lightly tap the breast
in a 'dancing' motion. Use a circular movement around

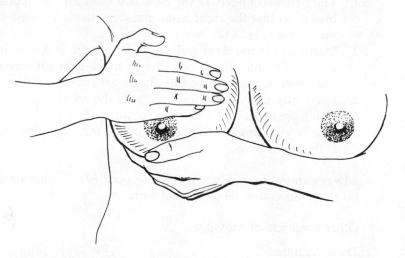

Fig. 3.13 *Alternative methods of breast massage – using both hands.*

the breast, or move the fingers from the edges of the breast to the areola in straight lines, gradually working all around the breast (see Fig. 3.14).

- Use a comb to stroke the breast gently from the edges of the breast to the areola.

3.7 Supplementary and replacement (complementary) feeding

A term, healthy baby should require no supplementary feeds (i.e. no extra fluids in addition to feeding from the breast); the baby should be fed on demand. Night feeds are particularly important and a baby should be given to the mother to breastfeed rather than be given a replacement (complementary) feed (i.e. a total feed in place of feeding from the breast), so that she can sleep. Only if there is a very good medical reason for not waking her should demand breastfeeding be interrupted.

Term babies admitted to a neonatal unit, who are capable of feeding on demand, come into this category. They include:

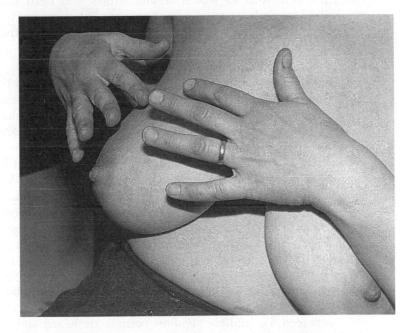

Fig. 3.14 *Alternative methods of breast massage – using the fingertips.*

- Babies receiving antibiotic therapy or phototherapy.
- Low birthweight babies (i.e. less than 2500 g at birth), who are awake and hungry, with a satisfactory blood sugar level.

There is no reason for these babies to have replacement feeding or supplementary feeding.

Giving supplementary or replacement feeds can lead to the mother's own milk supply decreasing. This also applies where rigid timing between feeds does not allow a baby to feed when ready, particularly if formula milk is used as the supplement. If a baby is hungry, the breast should be given, even if this is not at the times scheduled on a feeding chart. In hot weather, there is no evidence that supplementary feeding is necessary. Breastfeeding provides sufficient fluid for a term baby's needs.[23]

3.7.1   When supplementary or replacement feeds are necessary

There are situations in which certain babies will need supplementary or replacement feeds. These are listed below. It is preferable to use a mother's own expressed milk, rather than a formula milk.

1. If a baby is preterm and unable to take a full feed from the breast he will require supplementary feeding via a nasogastric or orogastric tube or cup. This usually applies to a baby who is just beginning to learn to breastfeed and only suckles for a very short time. As the baby becomes more efficient at the breast, less milk will need to be given by tube or cup and fewer supplementary feeds will be needed.

   It is impossible to suggest a regime which is suitable in all cases because each individual baby is so different. Some preterm or sick babies will breastfed well on one occasion in the day and require no supplementary feeds, while the same baby on another occasion will feed only for a few minutes and need a supplement. Some babies will not feed again for the rest of the day and require complete replacement feeds. If a well preterm baby has taken a satisfactory breast feed, i.e. audible swallow sounds are heard and the mother's breasts are comfortable after the feed, and her baby settles well afterwards, a supplement should not be necessary. Similarly, if the baby wakes and appears hungry after $1\frac{1}{2}$–2 hours, the breast should be offered again before any attempt at supplementation is made.

The mother should be encouraged to express her breastmilk so that she has some milk in the refrigerator or freezer, which can be used for a supplementary or replacement feed. If a baby goes to the breast for part of a feed the mother should express both breasts afterwards. This milk can then be used for the next feed if required.

2. A very sleepy jaundiced baby may need supplementation via a nasogastric or orogastric tube, or a cup, if regular breastfeeds are not possible. This is usually only necessary for a very short time. The mother should express during this period, but the baby should always be offered the breast before supplementation. Unless the jaundiced baby is also preterm, replacement feeds are unlikely to be required.

3. Supplementation or replacement feeding of a sick baby, whether term or preterm, may be required until the baby is strong or well enough to sustain his nutritive needs totally from the breast. The baby should be held next to the breast when ever possible so that, if he does want to breastfeed, he has the opportunity; a gastric tube feed can be given at the same time. The mother should be reassured that once a sick baby is better, feeding from the breast will improve. Similarly, if the baby is preterm, as he matures his feeding will also improve. The mother may need to be very patient.

In any situation where a supplement is considered necessary but there is insufficient expressed breast milk, always try to mix some mother's milk with the formula milk – this enhances the digestion of the formula milk.

Always make sure supplementary feeds are necessary!

3.8 Breast shells/drip catchers

These should only be used to catch drip milk at the time of feeding. If worn between feeds, they can create pressure on the lactiferous sinuses, and cause subsequent blockage and mastitis.

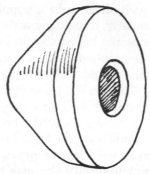

Fig. 3.15 *A breast shell.*

There is no evidence to show that breast shells (Fig. 3.15) improve the protractibility of a flat or inverted nipple in the antenatal period.[23]

References

1   Lang S, Lawrence CJ and L'E Orme R (1994) Sodium in hand and pump expressed human breast milk. *Early Hum Dev* **38**: 131–138.
2   World Health Organization (1989) Infant feeding: the physiological basis. *Bulletin* **67** (Suppl.): 76–77.
3   Hopkinson JM, Schanler RJ and Garza C (1988) Milk production by mothers of preterm infants. *Pediatrics* **81**: 815–819
4   Marmet C (1985) *Manual Expression of Breast Milk – Marmet Technique*. Reprint no. 27. Franklin Park, IL: Le Leche League International.
5   Mathur NB, Dwarkadas AM, Sharma VK *et al.* (1990) Anti-infective factors in preterm human colostrum. *Acta Paediatr Scand* **79**: 1039–1044.
6   Jannson L, Karlson FA and Westermark B (1985) Mitogenic activity and epidermal growth factor content in human milk. *Acta Paediatr Scand* **74**: 250–253.
7   Cure in a mother's milk. *New Scientist* 20 April, 1991.
8   Zinaman MJ, Hughes V, Queenan JT *et al.* (1992) Acute prolactin and oxytocin responses and milk yields to infant suckling and artificial methods of expression in lactating women. *Pediatrics* **89**: 437–440.
9   Auerbach KG (1990) Sequential and simultaneous breast pumping: a comparison. *Int J Nutrition Stud* **27**: 257–265.
10 Howie PJ, McNeilly AS, McArdle T *et al.* (1980) The relationship between suckling-induced prolactin response and lactogenesis. *J Clin Endocrinol Metabol* **50**: 670–673.
11 La Leche League International (1992) *The Breastfeeding Answer Book*. Franklin Park, IL: Le Leche League International, Ch. 4.
12 Jensen R and Jenson G (1992) Speciality lipids for infant nutrition.

1. Milks and formulas'. *J Pediatr Gastroenterol Nutrition* **15**: 232–245.

13   Pittard WB, Anderson DM, Cerutti ERC and Boxerbaum B (1985) Bacteriological qualities of human milk. *J Pediatr* **107**: 240–243.

14   Ellis L and Hamosh M (1991) Human milk: Stability of digestive enzymes in expressed milk. In *Human Lactation V: Mechanisms Regulating Lactation and Infant Nutrient Utilisation.* Picciano MF, Lonnerdal B (eds). Chichester: J Wiley and Sons, pp. 389–393.

15   Hopkinson J, Garza C and Asquith MT (1990) Human milk storage in glass containers. *H Human Lactation* **6**: 104–105.

16   Sigman M, Burke KL and Swarner OW (1989) Effects of microwaving human milk: Changes in IgA content and bacterial count. *J Am Diet Assoc* **89**: 690–692.

17   Lammi-Keefe CJ, Ferris AM and Jensen RG (1990) Changes in human milk at 0600, 1000, 1400, 1800, and 2200 h. *J Pediatr Gastroenterol Nutrition* **11**: 83–88.

18   Sosa R and Barness L (1987) Bacterial growth in refrigerated human milk. *Am J Dis Child* **141**: 111–112.

19   Minami J (1985) Helping mothers with Letdown. Oregon Areas Leaders' letter of La Leche League.

20   Riordan J (1989) *A Practical Guide to Breastfeeding.* Boston: Jones & Bartlett, pp. 262–273.

21   Bose CL, D'Ercole J, Lester AG, *et al.* (1981) Relactation by mothers of sick and preterm infants. *Pediatrics* **67**: 565–569.

22   De Carvalho M, Klaus MH and Merkatz RB (1982) Frequency of breast-feeding and serum bilirubin. *Am J Dis Child* **136**: 737–738.

23   The MAIN Trial Collaborative Group (1994) Preparing for breastfeeding: treatment of inverted and non-protractile nipples in pregnancy. *Midwifery* **10**: 200–211.

4 Breast conditions

4.1 How to cope with engorgement

4.1.1 Initial fullness of the breast

Fullness of the breast in the first few days after delivery is normal, and commonly occurs between 24 and 72 hours after delivery. It can be relatively mild and pass almost unnoticed, or severe and accompanied by a lot of pain and discomfort. This fullness is caused not only by the volume of milk increasing over a comparatively short time, but also by the venous system adjusting to hormonal changes. It should settle within 24–48 hours. All mothers, whether they breast- or bottle-feed will experience some degree of fullness.[1] Reassure mothers who are bottle-feeding using a formula milk that, as long as they do not stimulate their breasts or remove the breastmilk, the discomfort will pass. A firm, well-fitting brassiere may help at this time.

The second or third day after delivery is commonly a time when a mother may feel tearful and emotional. If the baby is also in a neonatal or paediatric unit, or has anything wrong with him, the mother's emotions may be even more labile. It is important, therefore, that she avoids preventable breast conditions which may interfere with her ability to feed her baby.

Although there is no 'cure' for venous engorgement, for it is self-limiting, some of the practical advice which follows may help relieve some of the discomfort. If milk engorgement can be avoided, this will certainly help.

It is useful to tell a mother about breast fullness in the first few days post-delivery **before** it occurs. Practical advice should include some or all of the following as appropriate:

1. If the baby is term and able to feed without any problem, feeding him whenever he is hungry (demand feeding) will

relieve the fullness created by the milk. The feeds should not be timed in length.

2. If expression of milk is necessary use a mechanical or hand pump, or hand express regularly, at least 3 hourly. **Do not** leave long intervals between expressions. This will only increase breast fullness and may cause milk engorgement. Advise the mother, if she is uncomfortable in the night, to express or her breasts will feel much fuller in the morning.

3. If breast fullness is very uncomfortable, relief may be provided in the following ways:

   - Bathing the breasts in warm or hot water in a bowl, bath or shower, and expressing enough milk for the breasts to be comfortable, or allowing any milk to drain naturally.
   - Covering the breasts with a warm/hot towel and gently massaging and hand expressing.

4. Use clean washed cabbage leaves[2,3] (smooth, dark green leaves) to place around the breasts, making sure a hole is left for the nipple! This is very comforting if the leaves have just come from a refrigerator. Support the leaves inside a brassiere. It is thought that a substance in the leaves reduces oedema and improves milk flow. This is useful for both venous and milk fullness, engorgement, and for mastitis – and is guaranteed to bring a smile to the afflicted at a difficult time! Prolonged use of the leaves is believed to reduce milk flow,[2] therefore, the leaves should not be used for longer than is necessary to relieve the symptoms.

5. Take a mild analgesic for pain if necessary.

Reassure the mother that breast fullness is normal in the first few days and will last a short time only. If the nipples become flattened because of breast fullness, expression of a little milk by hand or with a hand pump before feeding will draw out the nipple, and soften the breast sufficiently to aid the baby to suckle.

4.1.2 Milk engorgement

Milk engorgement will occur when the breasts are not efficiently drained. It can happen at any time during lactation, particularly in the early days of breastfeeding, and like fullness, it can affect the whole of the breasts. It can be avoided by using the advice given for full breasts. If engorgement is not relieved, it may lead to mastitis.

Engorgement that affects particular lobes of the breast may also be caused by:

- Inefficient drainage of all or some of the functioning lobes of the breast during each feed. This can result from incorrect attachment and positioning of the baby.
- Irregular or long periods of time between feeds/ expression of milk.

4.2   Cracked and sore nipples

These are best avoided! The majority of cases of cracked and sore nipples are usually the result of incorrect positioning and attachment of the baby at the breast. Therefore, if this problem is experienced by a mother, the first and most important action is to make absolutely certain that the baby **is** correctly attached at the breast in a position that can be comfortably maintained throughout the feed. Ensure also that the mother knows the basic principles of attachment and can position her baby correctly herself.

Cracked and sore nipples may also be caused by:

- 'Nipple' feeding, rather than breastfeeding.
- The baby licking or biting the nipple.
- Mechanical/hand pumps.
- The baby being 'pulled' off the breast when attached, without the seal around the breast being broken first.
- Infections, such as thrush (*Candida albicans*), which will require medical treatment to both the mother and baby.

There is no evidence to suggest that fair-skinned mothers are more likely to suffer sore/cracked nipples than any other mothers.

4.2.1   Sore nipples (pink/red with no cracks)

If a mother has sore nipples, with no cracks, suggest the following measures.

At the time of feeding

- Begin the milk flow before putting the baby to the breast, i.e. hand express a little milk on to the nipple.
- Some mothers find it helpful to begin the feed on the unaffected or less sore side first. The vigorous suckling action that some of them experience at the start of a feed is then gentler when the baby is attached to the breast with the sore nipple.
- Attach and position the baby correctly. If pain continues, reposition the baby and reattach him.
- To remove the baby from the breast, the mother should slide her little finger into the baby's mouth. This breaks the seal he has made with his lips around the areola/breast.
- Some mothers may find that giving the baby 10–15 ml of breastmilk before the feed begins helps to reduce the initial vigour of the baby's suck, particularly if the baby is very hungry.
- A nipple shield is seldom of any use in this situation. If one is used, the mother should be aware this is a **temporary solution only**. Nipple shields may be a cause of sore or cracked nipples if they do not fit exactly because they cause stress to the delicate area at the junction of the nipple and areola.

Between feeds or expressing

- Remove brassiere and breast pads until the nipples are healed. (If the mother finds it uncomfortable without a brassiere, suggest she wears either a cotton stretch cropped top (see Fig. 4.1) or supports her breasts with a cotton scarf loosely tied around her body (see Fig. 4.2).
- Some mothers may find expressing a little milk on to the nipple and smoothing it around the sore area helps the healing process, although there is little research to show that this works.
- Keep the breasts exposed to the air or under loose clothing, preferably made of a natural fibre, such as cotton.

No other treatment is usually necessary.

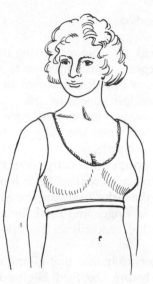

Fig. 4.1 *A comfortable support for the breasts – a cropped top.*

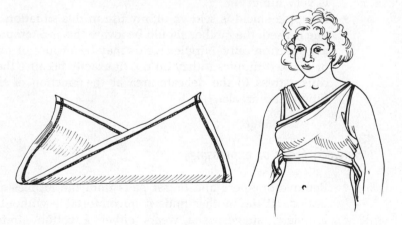

Fig. 4.2 *A comfortable support for the breasts – a cotton scarf.*

4.2.2   Nipples that are cracked and sore

Follow the above advice paying particular attention to the correct attachment and positioning of the baby. Assure the mother that the cracks, although very painful, will heal very quickly.
    In addition:

1. If the cracks in the nipple make it too painful to feed, use the unaffected side only (if possible).

2. Hand express 3 hourly from the affected breast to drain it regularly and avoid engorgement. Hand/mechanical pumps can make cracks worse. However, some mothers may find using pumps acceptable. The expressed milk is quite safe to give to the baby, unless it is heavily contaminated with blood (which may cause the baby to vomit).
3. If both the nipples are painful, gently hand express to start the milk flow and then attach the baby at the breast.

Apart from breast milk itself, there is some anecdotal evidence that geranium leaves give 'instant relief, if the furry side is placed on the nipple'![4] Some mothers may also find certain preparations, such as Calendula cream, vitamin E preparations or refined lanolin work for them, but it is not **necessary** for mothers to use these.

If a mother finds the pain from a sore/cracked nipple seriously interferes with breastfeeding, she can express her breastmilk and 'rest' her breasts for one or more feeds. She can give her milk to her baby by cup, or by gastric tube if this is considered appropriate. Once her breasts feel more comfortable she can resume breastfeeding.

4.3   Inverted and flat nipples (Figs 4.3 and 4.4)

The shape of a mother's nipples should not adversely affect her success at breastfeeding. However, an inverted or flat nipple

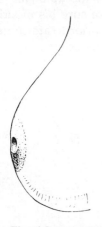

Fig. 4.3 *An inverted nipple.*   **Fig. 4.4** *A flat nipple.*

shape may make it more difficult for the baby to be well attached at the breast, and in the initial period of establishing breastfeeding the mother may require extra help.

If inverted or flat nipples have been observed in the antenatal period, the shape may improve after delivery when protractility of the nipple is more likely to occur. This may be particularly noticeable after suckling. It is important to emphasize to the mother that the baby should be **breast**feeding not **nipple** feeding. Therefore, it is the position and attachment at the breast which is of crucial importance to the baby's success at breastfeeding.

4.3.1   Management of inverted or flat nipples

- Stimulation of the nipples to make them as erect as possible may help with both nipple shapes. This can be achieved by gently rolling and pulling the nipple out prior to breastfeeding.
- Ensure the area around the nipple and areola is soft prior to breastfeeding.
- Position the baby for feeding at the breast in such a way that attachment is made as easy as possible. One position to consider, for example, is to have the baby laying on his mother's lap so that she can lean over with her breast falling into the baby's mouth.
- Attach the baby to the breast, with his bottom lip on the underside of the areola aimed as far away from the junction of the nipple and areola as possible. His top lip or his nose should be in line with the nipple. Make sure his mouth is opened as widely as possible (Fig. 4.5) prior to attachment. Bring him quickly to the breast once this occurs.

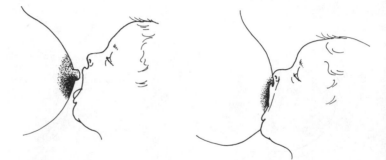

Fig. 4.5 *Attachment of a baby at the breast.*

- Use a breast reliever or a breast pump to soften the nipple, and encourage the nipple to become more prominent.
- A 10 or 20 ml syringe can also be used to help draw the nipple out just before a feed[5] (Fig. 4.6):

   (a) Cut approximately 3 cm off the nozzle end off the syringe.

   (b) Remove the plunger and insert it into the cut end.

   (c) Place the smooth end of the syringe barrel over the nipple.

   (d) Pull the plunger out. Be very **gentle**. Maintain the pressure applied.

   (e) The nipple should be drawn into the barrel.

   (f) To remove the syringe from the breast, push the plunger in, to release the suction.

This treatment can be used for 30 seconds to 1 minute, several times in the day. However, if any pain is felt during the process, it is important to push the plunger in and

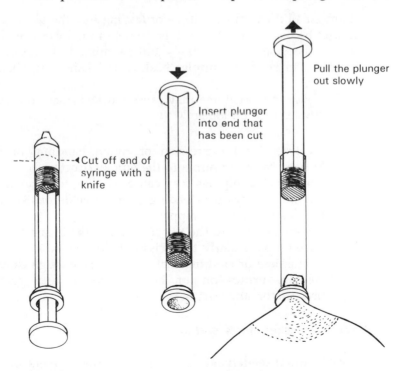

Pull the plunger out slowly

Insert plunger into end that has been cut

◀ Cut off end of syringe with a knife

Fig. 4.6 *The syringe method of treating inverted nipples.*

release the suction created. This will prevent any damage occurring to the nipple or the areola.

No device for treating inverted nipples should be left in place for any longer than is necessary to draw the nipple out (a few seconds in most cases).

- **Do not** make negative comments to the mother about her nipple shape.

4.4   Blocked ducts, lobes, mastitis and breast abscess

All of these are best avoided. The advice contained at the beginning of this chapter and in Chapter 2 (positioning and attachment) will certainly help prevent these conditions.

4.4.1   Blocked ducts and lobes

If any small ducts in the nipple or leading into the lactiferous sinuses become blocked and milk cannot drain, lobes can very quickly become uncomfortably full of milk. It is essential, therefore, to keep the nipples healthy and handle the breast correctly.

The following situations may cause blocked ducts and subsequently lead to full lobes:

- Incorrect hand expression or rough handling of the breasts, causing trauma to the nipples/ducts.
- Sore, cracked nipples may cause swelling to occur in or around the tiny ducts leading from the lactiferous sinuses to the surface of the nipple.
- Compression from the fingers holding the breast during a feed – particularly the 'scissor' hold (Fig. 4.7).
- A brassiere or clothing that is not loose enough during feeding, expression or between feeds, and causes pressure on any part of the breast.

Signs of blocked ducts and lobes

- Unusual tenderness or hardness in one segment of the breast. The outline of any underlying lump often follows

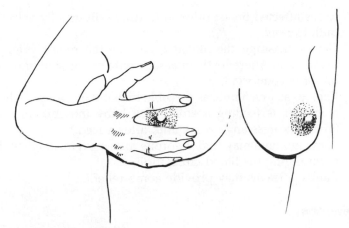

Fig. 4.7 *The 'scissor' hold.*

the margins of a lobe (more than one lobe may be affected if a duct in the nipple is blocked).
- A patch of red skin often appears over the hard area.

Treatment

Treatment is aimed at restoring the milk flow as soon as possible, otherwise mastitis will develop and, if this is not properly treated, an abscess may form. This can happen **very quickly**, within 24–48 hours. Advise the mother to continue breastfeeding. If she stops the problem will be made worse!

The suggested treatment is as follows:

1. Feed the baby whenever he is willing to suckle. Try not to have long gaps between feeds, especially during the acute phase of the condition. This may mean expressing the breastmilk if the baby does not want to suckle regularly.
2. Assess the baby's attachment at the breast and improve this if necessary, so that all the lactiferous sinuses are drained efficiently. Leaning forward will help drain the breasts if they are heavy or pendulous. A small rolled towel or flannel placed under the breast will help to enhance drainage of the lobes. Make sure that the baby's position is stable and not likely to affect his correct attachment. Feed him from both breasts if possible.
3. A bath or shower, or application of a warm flannel or towel

to the affected breast prior to feeding will usually help the milk to flow.

4. Gently massage the affected part of the breast prior to expression. Alternate the massage with expression until the breast is comfortable.
5. Express as much milk as possible by hand or pump. (Where a mother is feeding a small/sick baby intermittently by breast, express any excess milk after a feed.)
6. Some mothers may find vigorous arm movements help, by encouraging the blood circulation.
7. Cabbage leaves may provide some relief.

Prevention

1. Feed on demand.
2. Avoid tight clothing.
3. Correct positioning and attachment of the baby during a breastfeed.
4. If expressing, use a 2–3 hourly regime.
5. If a baby has an eye infection, make sure it is cleaned prior to breastfeeding.

4.4.2 Mastitis

This will develop if a blocked duct is not treated promptly. In approximately 50% of cases, it is non-infective[6] and will respond to the treatment given in the above section. **Do not give up breastfeeding.** The problem or infection is in the breast tissue, not the milk. The inflammation and pain that may accompany mastitis is caused by the milk being forced out of the alveoli into the surrounding breast tissue. This causes a localized and acute inflammatory reaction to occur. It is sometimes difficult without culturing the milk to know if an infection is also present. In both infective or non-infective mastitis the initial treatment is exactly the same.

Signs of mastitis

- Painful breasts.
- A hot, red swelling – often following the shape of one or two lobes.

- There may be fever and flu-like symptoms, e.g. aching, lethargy.

Treatment

1. As already described for blocked lobes and ducts.
2. Start each feed from the affected side, if possible. Gently massage the breast before/during the feed.
3. If the mother is feverish, make sure she does not become dehydrated.
4. Encourage the mother to rest, and get someone else to do the shopping, cooking and cleaning.
5. Apply hot and/or cold compresses to the affected area between feeds, whichever is most comfortable.
6. **Remember the cabbage leaves**, especially if they are just taken out of a refrigerator – they may help soothe the breast.
7. Give analgesia to the mother, if required.
8. If pain or inflammation continues, despite the advice so far given, a doctor must be consulted promptly. Antibiotics may be necessary. However, **breastfeeding should be continued**. Antibiotics may cause diarrhoea in the baby, who may then require more frequent feeding. This will usually help relieve the mastitis more quickly and will not harm the baby.
9. **Drainage of the milk is vital**, however it is achieved. If there is still discomfort after feeding, then expression with a pump or by hand is necessary. Hand expression may be more comfortable.

4.4.3 Breast abscess

These may form superficially, often near to the areola, or they may develop in the deeper tissue as a result of unresolved mastitis or abrupt weaning.

Signs of breast abscess

- A hard lump, which does not go away. It may **not** be painful.
- A generalized feeling of being unwell.
- A fever, which may be quite extreme and sudden.

Treatment

1. Prompt medical intervention is essential.
2. Treat any mastitis quickly using the advice in the above sections.
3. Continue feeding from the unaffected breast.
4. Milk from the affected breast should be expressed by pump or hand. This needs to be done as gently as possible to avoid any further trauma to the tissues.
5. If the abscess requires surgical drainage, breastfeeding should be commenced on the affected side as soon as possible, unless the incision site makes this impossible.
6. The mother will probably require advice on relactation to increase milk production on the affected side.

Remember **prevention is better than cure!** Treat any predisposing factor as it occurs.

4.5 Breastfeeding and nipple shields

Nipple shields (Fig. 4.8) **should not** be used without a very good reason. There is convincing evidence to suggest they can inhibit milk production, as stimulation of the nipple and breast is considerably reduced.[7] They are totally unsuitable for long-term use without specialist advice and, when they are used, they should be dispensed with as soon as possible.

Once a baby is used to feeding with a shield, it is extremely difficult to get him to breastfeed without it. The shield is used because a problem exists. It is important, therefore, before being tempted to use one, to assess the problem and see if a solution can be found, which avoids its use. The short-term gains of using a nipple shield may prove to be much more troublesome and time consuming in the long term. The fact that a baby is feeding 'well' with a shield does not mean the 'problem' has been solved. Its use is likely to adversely affect the mother's chances of establishing breastfeeding, unless considerable care is taken.

4.5.1 How to avoid the use of nipple shields

1. Teach mothers how to hand express:

    *   To avoid sore nipples.

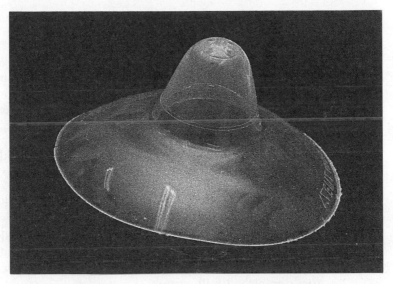

Fig. 4.8 *A nipple shield.*

- To start the milk flow at the beginning of the feed.
- To express directly into the baby's mouth.

2. Ensure the baby is positioned and attached correctly and appropriately for his size and gestation.
3. If the mother's nipples are flat or inverted, teach her to:

- Gently massage the nipples, to make them become more erect.
- Use a hand pump or breast reliever prior to the feed, to draw the nipple out, or to soften the breast, if it is engorged.
- Some mothers suggest using cold water or ice to make the nipples erect.

4. If the baby 'fights' at the breast:

- Feed the baby expressed breast milk by cup until he calms down.
- Use the nursing supplementer.
- Avoid using a bottle teat, dummy or nipple shield. All of these may give a baby who is to be breastfed an inappropriate experience of sucking. Sucking on a finger is likely to be of a shorter duration than using a dummy or nipple shield, but this **may also confuse** a

baby if it occurs frequently. All of these sucking devices may cause him to refuse to suckle correctly at the breast.

If, after trying to overcome the 'problem', it is still thought necessary, by either the mother or professional adviser, to use a nipple shield, make sure the mother is aware of the following points:

- Less suction will be felt than when the baby is suckling directly from the breast (the tip of the shield can be cut off to help alleviate this).
- The shield is only a **temporary** measure. It is not a permanent solution to the original problem.
- Continuous use of a shield may compromise the baby's weight gain. This is because decreased breast stimulation causes a reduction in the milk production, which leads to a diminished milk supply.
- If the mother wishes/insists on using a nipple shield when her baby leaves the hospital, make sure that she is followed up by the health visitor or the health professional who has been advising her in hospital or a breastfeeding counsellor. The baby will require regular weighing, either by returning to the hospital unit or to the local health centre.
- She must only use the thin **silicone** nipple shields. These come in two sizes. The smaller size frequently provides a better fit, though neither size is really satisfactory.

4.5.2 Situations in which a nipple shield may be appropriate

- A truly inverted, non-protractile nipple, if all else has consistently failed.
- Extremely traumatized nipples, where a mother **does not** wish to rest and express her breasts. In this case, correct advice on how to position and attach the baby is of paramount importance as well as advice on how to deal with her sore nipples. The nipple shield should be discontinued as soon as possible because it will only add to her problems.
- A baby with a cleft lip and/or palate, if her mother does not have protractile nipples. However, this should be used as a last resort, because this mother may not get

sufficient breast stimulation without a shield and will receive even less with one.
*   Too much milk.

Never use a nipple shield when a baby, term or preterm, is first learning to breastfeed (i.e. in the first few days after delivery, or after several days or weeks if the baby is unable to breastfeed at birth) – they are not a substitute for teaching correct positioning or attachment.

4.5.3 How to use nipple shields

*   Only use the thin silicon nipple shields (use the smaller size initially).
*   Always hand express a little milk into the nipple shield prior to the feed.
*   Make sure the shield fits the mother's nipple as closely as possible.
*   At the end of the feed, make sure there is evidence of milk in the shield.

4.5.4 How to wean a baby off the shield

There is no right or wrong way to wean a baby off a nipple shield. The method depends upon the baby and, to a great extent, the determination of the mother – and the support and help of the professional staff. It is also dependent on what the original problem was, the strategy adopted to solve it, and how often the shield has been and is being used.

When the shield has been used only once or twice:

1. Make sure the baby is positioned and attached at the breast correctly.
2. Hand express some milk on to the nipple.
3. Ensure the baby opens his mouth widely before he latches on to the nipple and areola.
4. Hand expressing directly into the baby's mouth initially may help.
5. If the baby is a healthy, term 'well-padded' baby, do not even consider using the nipple shield again – even if the baby complains bitterly! If the shield is given, the situation will just get more difficult and traumatic to correct. It is

better to have a short period of agitation than risk the mother's milk supply long term. When the baby is hungry enough, he will take the breast!

If the baby continues to refuse the breast:

6. Advise the mother to take her baby to bed with her for 24 hours, so that he gets plenty of opportunity to feed from the breast whenever he is hungry or thirsty.
7. Encourage as much skin to skin contact as possible, especially prior to feed times.

Where the shield has been used for 1–2 days or longer, or where it has been used with a small or underweight baby, the method may be less straight forward:

1. If the mother and baby are relaxed at the beginning of the feed, try using the above methods first. If, however, after 5–10 minutes there is no success, use the nipple shield.
2. Alternatively use the shield for a fraction of the feed. For example, if a feed normally takes 15 minutes, use the shield for 5 minutes. Then try to attach the baby at the breast when the milk is flowing well and the breast tissue soft.
3. As already suggested, encourage the mother to have a day in bed with her baby and encourage skin-to-skin contact as often as possible.
4. Use the nursing supplementer.
5. Fill a syringe with expressed breastmilk, and squeeze a little milk on to the nipple or areola just before the baby is offered the breast. This is useful when the mother is very tense and her milk is not flowing easily.

References

1   Parazzini F, Zanaboni F, Liberati A and Tognoni G (1989) Breast symptoms in women who are not breastfeeding. In *Effective Care in Pregnancy and Childbirth*. Enkin M, Keirse M, Chalmers I, (eds). Oxford: Oxford University Press, pp. 1390–1403.
2   Rosier W (1989) Cool cabbage compresses. *Breastfeeding Rev* (NMA, Nunawading, Victoria, Australia), November.
3. Nikodem VC, Danziger D, Gebka N, Gulmezoglu AM and Hofmeyer J (1993) Do cabbage leaves prevent breast engorgement? A randomised, controlled study. *Birth* **20**: 61–64.

4.   Lloyd J (1992) Now geraniums?? *Australian Lactation Consultants Assoc News* **3** (August): 3–4.
5.   WHO/UNICEF (1993) *Breastfeeding Counselling: A Training Course* Secretariat, Division of Diarrhoeal and Acute Respiratory Disease Control, Session 14, pp. 194–195. WHO, Geneva, Switzerland.
6.   *Royal College of Midwives* (1991) Antenatal and postnatal considerations. In *Successful Breastfeeding*, 2nd edn. London: Churchill Livingstone, pp. 53–59.
7   Woolridge M, Baum D and Drewitt RF (1980) Effect of a traditional and of a new nipple shield on sucking patterns and milk flow. *Early Human Development* **4**: 357–364.

5 The milk supply

5.1 Too little milk

There are several causes for a low milk production and sub-sequently a low milk supply. Usually it is a combination of factors which are responsible. Only 3–4% of mothers have a genuine breastmilk insufficiency,[1] caused by a lack of functioning glandular tissue. Mothers with babies on a neonatal or paediatric unit commonly experience a fluctuating milk supply. This appears to be related to the 'ups and downs' of their baby's medical condition. Periods of acute stress usually coincide with a temporary reduction in the mother's milk supply, and this can make a mother even more anxious, causing her to worry about her apparent low milk volume on expression. Thus, a vicious circle can be created very quickly. The mother requires constant reassurance and support. Once she is aware that a temporary inhibition of her 'let down' reflex may occur at times it is easier for her to cope with this reaction to her baby's condition. Many mothers who experience this temporary fluctuation do not appear to suffer any permanent reduction in their milk supply – as long as they continue to express regularly.

During the first 2 or 3 months after delivery, there may be times when the milk supply seems inadequate for a 24–48 hour period. The baby may become irritable and want to feed more frequently. This is quite **normal** and usually coincides with the baby having a period of rapid growth.[2] Once the mother's body adjusts to her baby's new requirements, the baby's feeding regime returns to how it was before. Unless a mother knows this is one of the events that can normally occur during lactation, she may think her milk supply is beginning to diminish. It is not uncommon for mothers to experience this at around the 5 or 6 week period – which coincides with one of the time periods when mothers often give up breastfeeding.[3]

5.1.1   Physical factors that may interfere with, or cause low milk production

- The possibility of retained placenta should be suspected, if the milk supply is difficult to initiate in the first few days following delivery.[4] It is always worth checking the mother's notes to see if the placenta was complete at delivery. Any large blood clots passed should be reported to and examined by the maternity staff.
- Inverted nipples can be an indication that the mother has a reduced number of lobes in the breast, which may result in a reduced output of milk.[5] In this case it is important for the mother to be given all the information from this section. She should be encouraged to produce as much milk as she can, so that it can be used in conjunction with any formula milk the baby may also receive.
- Breast surgery, in which either the lobes, the ductal system or the nerve supply have been partially removed or damaged will affect the milk production.
- Low maternal thyroid level.[6]

Any milk a mother expresses is valuable.

Mothers who have a low milk supply, for which none of the above factors is thought to be responsible, may find some of the following suggestions helpful. Mothers with a genuine problem of milk production will also benefit from some of these suggestions aimed at optimizing their milk supply, though this may continue to result in a low milk output and the baby may still require supplementation with a formula milk or human banked milk.

5.1.2   Suggested remedies

1. Feed the baby on demand, even if this means more frequently than is indicated on his fluid chart (as long as he is not fluid restricted). This will help build up the mother's milk production and supply.
2. If the mother is in a 'mother and baby room' and her baby is able to breastfeed without any problem, advise her to take her baby to bed with her, so that she can feed him whenever required. This is possible if her baby is begin-

ning to learn to breastfeed or breastfeeding is already well established.

3. A mother needs to have sufficient rest, both during the day and at night.

4. Before feeding or expressing, she should try to sit down for 5-10 minutes (longer if possible!) with a warm drink and with some favourite music – preferably restful! She may find that gently massaging her breasts, will help to relax her, thus improving her 'let-down' reflex.

5. Express from warm breasts in a warm room. If a mother is cold, advise her to have a warm bath or shower prior to massage and expression, or to bathe the breasts in warm water, or put a warm towel or flannel on the breasts prior to massaging and expression.

6. Make sure, if the mother is using a mechanical pump, that she massages for a few minutes prior to expression.

7. Observe her expressing with the pump to check her technique, make sure she is expressing for long enough, alternating between the breasts, and is expressing at least 6–8 times per day. If possible encourage her to express 2–3 hourly for 24–48 hours, i.e. 8–10 times. Advise her to express at least once in the night with no long intervals between sessions. If this is not successful, suggest the mother uses hand expression or a hand pump.

8. Advise the mother to express from both breasts **after** a feed. This is particularly important if the baby is preterm and has a weak suck, which may not stimulate the mother's milk production efficiently.

9. An alternative to the previous method of stimulating the milk supply is to let the mother express her milk for 24–48 hours and, after each expression, encourage the baby to suck on the *emptied breast*.[7] The baby can be given milk either by cup or oral gastric tube. This may also be a useful method for a preterm baby, who needs practice at the breast, but is still receiving most of his feeds by tube.

10. The nursing supplementer can help build up the milk supply by encouraging the baby to suckle and, therefore, provides stimulation of the breast.

11. The mother may need to rethink her priorities. Housework, for example, may have to be given a secondary position for a while and offers of help should not be refused!

It may be impossible for her to have the same daily routines she had before she was pregnant.

12. If the mother has previously produced good volumes of milk, reassure her that she will again.

13. Advise the mother that, if her partner massages her breasts or otherwise stimulates them, this can have a very positive result. Either she or her partner can very gently massage her nipples, which encourages the release of prolactin and oxytocin.

14. Encourage the mother's partner or a friend to massage her back (see Section 3.4 'Prolonged expression of breastmilk').

15. Check any drugs that the mother may be taking. If she is a smoker, make sure that she smokes **after** feeding or expressing, not before.

16. Warn the mother that when she is discharged from hospital she may notice a temporary reduction in her milk supply, but she should continue to express as previously. The reduction may be a result of the mother not expressing as frequently or for as long as when she was in hospital.

17. Metoclopromide, domperidone in small doses, or oxytocin nasal spray (in some countries) are sometimes recommended to stimulate the milk supply, and are worth considering if other advice consistently fails.[8,9] These drugs would have to be prescribed by the mother's doctor.

18. Check whether the mother has resumed taking an oral contraceptive. Make certain she is on the mini-pill, which contains progesterone only. If she has been commenced on the combined pill, this will diminish her milk supply because of the effect of oestrogen.[10] In this case, tell the mother to contact her doctor immediately or, if necessary, you should contact her doctor to ensure she is prescribed the correct contraceptive drug. This may be one cause of a diminishing milk supply at around 6 weeks.

19. A homeopathic remedy for diminished milk supply is 'Mother tincture' (*Urtica urens*). This is obtainable from a homeopathic pharmacy. However, if a mother wishes to use homeopathic remedies it is important she consults a **registered homeopath**.[21] Acupuncture may also be worth considering, in which case it is important to consult a

registered acupuncturist. (The Appendix contains the addresses of the professional organizations from where locally registered practitioners can be obtained.)

Reassure the mother that a diminished milk supply is only a temporary problem.

5.2   Too much milk and leaking breasts

Having more breastmilk than is required may seem to be an advantage, but it can be a source of concern to mothers (particularly if the milk leaks on to her clothes, or her baby is supplemented with a formula milk even though she is expressing more milk than her baby needs). For the majority of mothers an abundant milk supply is not a permanent problem. If it continues beyond the first week after birth in a mother breastfeeding a healthy term baby, it usually suggests that incorrect attachment may be the cause. However, sometimes when a baby is breastfeeding for all or some of his feeds at around 33–36 weeks gestation or post-conception age, or he is weakened by illness, his mother may experience an abundant milk supply which continues beyond the first few days of lactation.

There are a number of ways to help a mother:

1. If the flow from the breast is too fast, owing to a forceful let-down reflex, the milk may fill the baby's mouth too quickly, causing him to choke and, therefore, 'fight' at the breast. In this case, it may help if the mother expresses some milk prior to feeding (20–30 ml is usually sufficient to slow the flow). This will also ensure that the mother is not left uncomfortably full at the end of a feed. In addition, it will enable the baby to obtain more of the fat-rich hindmilk, which will be more satisfying than a feed high in foremilk, and will ensure the baby has an adequate weight gain.
2. If the milk continues to come too fast, a different position for feeding may be beneficial. The flow may be slowed if the mother lies on her back or reclines in a chair, with her baby positioned on her abdomen, so he can easily take the breast. The baby's head can be supported with the mother's hand on his forehead (Fig. 5.1).

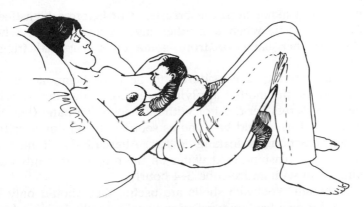

Fig. 5.1 *Positioning a baby when the mother has a very abundant milk flow.*

3. A nipple shield may be useful, as this is known to reduce the supply of milk.
4. It takes approximately 6 weeks to really establish breastfeeding, by which time this problem has usually resolved. It is important for a mother to know that it is not a permanent condition.
5. Hand expression reduces the amount of milk obtained if expression of breastmilk continues to be necessary.

Some mothers who have to express breastmilk for a baby in a neonatal or paediatric unit, and who choose to use a mechanical pump, may find that they are able to express volumes well in excess of their baby's needs. When expression has to be maintained for several weeks, the mother's milk production may still be very high when her baby is ready to breastfeed. Many mothers find that it takes several days for their milk production to adjust to the needs of the baby, rather than the pump (even when the mother is no longer using a pump). If this artificial stimulation is the probable cause of an excessive milk supply, the suggested ways of weaning a mother off a mechanical pump are appropriate (see Section 3.4.2 'How to stop using a pump').

5.2.1 Leaking breasts

This can also be very distressing to mothers. It does not occur because there is too much milk but because the tiny muscles in the nipple are weak. An over-enthusiastic let-down reflex can cause leaking from the breasts, at or before a breastfeed. This can occur when a mother hears her baby cry, when she sees her baby, or from some other personal trigger mechanism.

When leaking is considered to be a problem, it can be stopped by the mother applying pressure to the nipples with her arms across her chest or with the heel of her hand (Figs 5.2 and 5.3). This should be done as soon as the let-down or tingling sensation, or leaking is felt. Alternatively, it may be helped by splashing cold water on the nipples or gently rubbing them with an ice-cube 3–4 hourly.

Although Woolwich shells are useful, they should only be worn during a feed or expression to collect milk draining from the other breast, as they can encourage leaking by causing pressure on the milk sinuses.

Breast pads can be worn to absorb leaking milk, but should be abandoned if the nipples become sore or cracked, particularly if they are lined with plastic. Sometimes going without a brassiere and wearing loose clothing will help because there is less nipple stimulation.

This problem usually resolves itself within a few weeks. It is rarely a permanent condition.

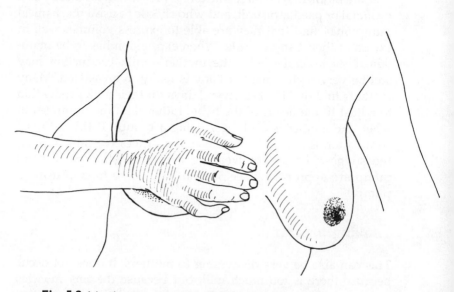

Fig. 5.2 *A hand position to prevent milk leakage.*

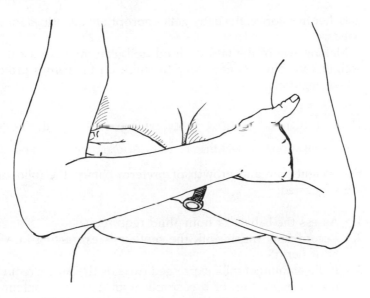

Fig. 5.3 *The position of the arms to prevent milk leakage.*

5.3   Expression of the fat-rich hind-milk

The quality of the milk given to a preterm, low birthweight or sick baby is of paramount importance to his growth and well-being. How a mother practically expresses may possibly influence the quality of her breastmilk, which is subsequently given to her baby. To optimize the collection of milk that is most beneficial to a baby, it is necessary to look at some very basic aspects of expression.

A baby requires a balanced diet of breastmilk, which contains adequate amounts of fore-milk, and of hind-milk, with its higher fat content. A problem may occur, however, if the mother has an abundant milk supply when expressing with an electric pump. The fat-rich hind-milk, containing valuable calories important to the baby's growth, may not be collected in a way which is easy to feed to him. If as a result growth begins to slow, a low birthweight or standard formula milk may be introduced to the baby's diet.

It is possible, if the mother has a sufficiently good milk supply, to express it in a way that ensures a balance of the fore- and hind-milk. Thus, the baby receives the benefit of the mother's milk without needing as much additional formula milk or fortification. It also has another advantage: because it is richer in calories, the baby gets appropriate quantities for his needs.

Making use of the fat-rich hind-milk can improve a baby's weight gain but it is necessary to check on the baby's protein intake regularly.[11]

5.3.1   Promotion of weight gain and growth in preterm babies

For weight gain and growth of preterm babies, the following are suggested:

1.   Assess the baby's 24 hour fluid requirements.
2.   Record how much milk the mother is expressing in a 24 hour period.
3.   If the amount of milk expressed exceeds the baby's requirements, expression of breastmilk with a higher content of the fat-rich hind-milk is possible.

5.3.2   The formula

The mother's total amount of expressed breastmilk produced in 24 hours, minus the baby's milk requirements.

Example

A mother produces 400 ml of breastmilk in 24 hours, and her baby requires 200 ml of milk in 24 hours. At each expression the mother needs to express approximately half of her milk from both breasts into 'Bottle 1', this containing higher levels of fore-milk, and the remainder from both breasts into 'Bottle 2', which will contain both fore- and hind-milk. The milk in 'Bottle 2' will be given to the baby. The milk in 'Bottle 1' will be refrigerated.

Baby's requirements = 200 ml/24 hours.
Mother's previous 24 hour total = 405 ml.

At each expression on the previous day the mother's totals were:

1.   Early morning = 80 ml

2. Mid-morning = 75 ml
3. Lunch time = 70 ml
4. Mid-afternoon = 65 ml
5. Early evening = 60 ml
6. Bedtime   = 55 ml

Therefore, the mother's regime for 'Bottle 1' should be:

1. 40 ml (20 + 20 ml)
2. 40 ml (20 + 20 ml)
3. 30 ml (15 + 15 ml)
4. 30 ml (15 + 15 ml)
5. 30 ml (15 + 15 ml)
6. 30 ml (15 + 15 ml)

All the remaining milk should be expressed into 'Bottle 2', which is then given to the baby.

Important points to remember when expressing

- Both breasts should be expressed for Bottle 1, and again for Bottle 2.
- The total amounts expressed into Bottle 1 and Bottle 2 will vary with each expression, although the proportions will be constant (see example). It is useful to look at the total quantity of milk produced at each expression on the previous day to provide a guide to the approximate amount to express into Bottle 1. The remainder of the milk can be expressed into Bottle 2.
- The bottles should be clearly labelled. Coloured labels are useful, not only are they easily seen and identifiable, but they are also easy for mothers to use. For example, if they are put in the freezer, a blue adhesive label could be attached to Bottle 1, and a yellow label to Bottle 2. The bottles with the yellow labels contain the richer milk and it is these that will be given to the baby.
- Ask the mother to keep a record of the amounts of milk she is expressing into Bottle 1 and Bottle 2.
- It is necessary to check the mother's milk supply daily. If it begins to diminish to a point where a surplus is no longer possible, **stop** expressing in this way and commence expressing the full amount into one bottle only, until there is an excess of milk again.

- Record on the baby's weight chart when feeding with the fat-rich hind-milk was commenced. Check on the baby's progress. If you have any worries about his growth or weight gain, please discuss it with the doctors.
- Write out the regime for the mother, so that she knows exactly what she must do and approximately how much she should express.

5.3.3 Promotion of weight gain in breastfeeding babies

If a mother has an adequate milk supply, but the weight gain of her baby is poor or static, and/or the baby is preterm or compromised by a clinical condition, expression of a quantity of fore-milk will ensure the baby is able to obtain milk containing the hind-milk during a breastfeed. The baby can then be offered the expressed fore-milk by cup if needed.

The amount of milk that should be expressed is as follows:

1. On day 1, express between 10 and 20 ml of fore-milk from each breast, before each breastfeed.
2. Breastfeed normally.
3. Give the expressed milk by cup, if the baby requires more after a breastfeed.
4. On days 2–5, express less milk prior to each breastfeed, until expressing is unnecessary.
5. If after this regime the weight gain begins to slow again, repeat the above regime.

As the baby matures this problem usually disappears.

5.4 The normal growth of the breastfed baby

A number of studies have shown that the growth patterns of breast- and formula-fed babies are different.[12–15] In the first 2 or 3 months after birth, breastfed babies put on weight more rapidly than formula-fed babies, but from the third or fourth months they tend to grow more slowly.[16–18] **This is normal.** Therefore, beware of current centile charts, they may not accurately reflect a breastfed baby's normal weight gain.

5.5   Weight loss and test weighing

A certain amount of weight loss is considered normal in the first few days of life. However, some term healthy babies born at home have been observed to have no initial weight loss,[19] possibly as a result of the the environment they were born into, i.e. a warm room, avoiding any initial heat loss, immediate and sustained skin-to-skin contact and access to the breast. Because the mothers were relaxed during labour and afterwards, it was suggested that larger volumes of colostrum may be produced. Colostrum has a higher osmotic pressure than mature milk, therefore, minimizing the initial water loss, which accounts for much of the initial weight loss at birth.[20,21] Babies who have a low birthweight for their gestational age are another group who may lose little weight at birth. These babies are often very hungry and may want to be fed more frequently than babies whose initial birthweight is appropriate for their gestational age.

By contrast among preterm babies, the lower the gestational age at birth the greater the initial weight loss is likely to be.

In a normal, term, healthy baby, birthweight is usually regained by the tenth day of life. If 10% or more of the birthweight is lost, it may be necessary to examine the possible causes, and particularly the method of feeding used.

5.5.1   Causes of weight loss

- Insufficient milk supply – this is a rare condition.
- The use of expressed breastmilk, which has a low fat content.
- A sleepy baby, not taking sufficient milk or not waking to feed on demand.
- Incorrect positioning and attachment at the breast.
- A preterm or sick baby lacking sufficient energy to feed long enough to obtain sufficient breastmilk or the hind-milk.

5.5.2   Test weighing

This is rarely necessary and may seriously undermine the mother's confidence.

The result of test weighing may totally misrepresent what the baby has taken in a breastfeed:

- The scales may not be accurate.
- The baby will almost certainly take different amounts at different feeds.
- There is no indication as to the nutritional value of the feed. A baby may have had 40 ml of fore- and hind-milk and be completely satisfied, or 50 ml of fore-milk and be totally unsettled – which weight would be accurate? More importantly, which baby will have had the most benefit from his feed?

If test weighing is considered necessary, it should be carried out over a 24 hour period. If it is the mother who wants the test weighing to be carried out, it is better to teach her how to recognize when her baby has had sufficient milk. If she still wishes her baby to be test weighed, the points above should be explained to her.

If it is the health professionals who want the baby to be test weighed, then the question 'why?' needs to be asked, to see if there is an alternative way to get the information required. Is it simply a lack of confidence in the mother's milk supply or her ability to meet her baby's requirements, or is it that health professionals feel more comfortable when they can count the number of ml the baby has taken, and know what the 'nutritional' quality of the milk is?

5.6   Breast surgery and feeding

Breast surgery **does not mean** that successful breastfeeding is impossible – except where bilateral mastectomy has been performed, or where the nipples have been removed or are absent. Successful breastfeeding is possible when:

- One breast has been removed but the other breast functions perfectly normally.
- The mother's nipples have been resited, but the nerves and ductal system have been left intact and can function in the different position.
- Breast reduction or silicon implant surgery has been performed, as long as the nerve supply of the nipple and the

ductal system necessary for lactation have been left intact (and the silicon implant is not leaking).
- Removal of breast lumps or drainage of a breast abscess has been performed.

It is necessary to read the mother's medical notes or to contact her general practitioner to discover exactly what treatment or surgery she has previously received, particularly in the case of major breast surgery.

In situations where surgery has reduced the milk supply temporarily, the nursing supplementer is invaluable, until the normal functioning of the breast returns. The mother may require advice and help with relactation.

In surgery where the normal functioning of the breast is no longer possible, providing the nipples are present, 'breastfeeding' can also be achieved using the nursing supplementer. A mother will need a lot of support and encouragement (as indeed will any mother who has undergone breast surgery – for whatever reason). The establishment of a satisfactory 'breastfeeding' technique using the nursing supplementer can be psychologically very beneficial to the mother and the relationship she has with her baby.

5.7 Relactation

Relactation is possible even if a mother has not breastfed for many months or even years, it is also possible to induce lactation in women who have never been pregnant.[22,23] However, it requires a commitment from the mother and a great deal of support from health professionals.

Relactation is useful for mothers of adopted babies, and where a baby in the neonatal unit has not been able to feed for many weeks and the mother's milk supply has diminished.

The stimulation required for a mother to produce breastmilk is of two kinds:

1. Mechanical, i.e. a pump, hand expression and a baby suckling.
2. Hormonal, i.e. if a mother has been pregnant in the past 6 months, her levels of oestrogen and progesterone may still be lower than before her pregnancy. Stimulation of the breasts may result in increases in prolactin (which produces

milk) and oxytocin (which makes milk available). If an adoptive mother has never been pregnant, she is likely to need hormonal preparations to induce breastmilk production.

5.7.1 Relactation if the mother has produced breastmilk previously

If the mother has a baby who is able to suckle:

1. Breastfeed the baby every 2 hours, throughout the night and day.
2. Allow the baby to suck as long as possible. Check on the baby's intake, weigh the nappies if they are very absorbent. Always weigh each nappy dry first, for each one may have a slightly different weight.
3. Supplementation will initially be required. Use a cup, spoon, syringe or the nursing supplementer where possible.
4. Continue this regime until milk can be hand expressed, and the baby is growing adequately without supplementation. Milk may begin to appear between 1 and 6 weeks after the stimulation and/or drug treatment begins.[24] An adequate milk supply may take several weeks to achieve.
5. Mothers may additionally require **metoclopramide**, 10 mg, three times a day, for at least 7 days. These drugs can only be obtained on a doctor's prescription.
6. Some mothers may also find additional breast stimulation from an electric pump is necessary.

If a mother has no opportunity of putting a baby to the breast:

1. A mother who has no baby to put to the breast may find she has sufficient stimulation from an electric pump to encourage the milk supply to build up, particularly if she has had a good milk supply in the past few weeks.
2. The mother should use a pump every 2 hours until she is able to express adequate volumes of milk for her baby's requirements, or until she is happy with the amounts expressed.
3. Treatment with metoclopramide should be considered.

5.7.2   Relactation if the mother has never produced breastmilk previously

1. All the advice given previously will help this mother.
2. Metoclopramide 10 mg, three times a day, together with frequent stimulation from the pump (10–12 times a day) may be necessary.[25]
3. Most mothers can produce sufficient volumes of milk to partially satisfy their baby's needs within 6 weeks of commencing treatment and pump stimulation.
4. The milk produced is considered to be equivalent to mature breastmilk.[26,27]

5.8   The mother's diet and fluids

Mothers tend to feel hungrier and thirstier during lactation and they will benefit if they eat when they feel hungry and drink when they feel thirsty!

Many mothers with babies on a neonatal or paediatric unit miss meals altogether, have no appetite or only have snacks when there is time and when they remember. While it is quite understandable that this should happen, a mother needs to take care of herself and may need gentle encouragement and persuasion to eat and drink regularly. Even though physiologically there may be no evidence to link diet with milk volume, a combination of stress, missed meals and a different routine appears to have the effect of temporarily reducing the mother's milk supply, possibly because she is not expressing as often as she needs to, or for as long at each session, thereby draining her breasts less effectively. If a mother is not given sufficient support at this time her milk production may be permanently affected as her confidence becomes undermined.

A balanced, healthy diet is ideal. It is essential, when giving advice to mothers, to find out what their normal diet and eating/drinking habits are, and to offer advice around this information, if necessary. A diet designed to lose weight is generally inappropriate for a lactating mother. Regular eating habits should be maintained with breakfast, a nutritious lunch and evening meal. Some mothers also find that they need a snack mid-morning, mid-afternoon and mid-evening. Some mothers prefer smaller more frequent meals during the day and evening, this is quite satisfactory and may have the advantage of ensuring an even caloric intake.

Many babies become more restless and are perceived to be more 'demanding' towards the evening. This may be because the mother's milk production is naturally lessened towards the end of the day. (Mothers who express milk will usually obtain more milk in the morning and less as the day proceeds.) Sometimes it helps a mother if she has a snack in the late afternoon and mid-evening. Small snacks of high caloric value can be beneficial in providing the body with sustainable energy to produce milk, e.g. halva, 'Build ups', dried fruits and cheese, appear to be useful. In addition it will greatly benefit the mother if she can have practical help with any tasks which have to be done in the evenings, for example, cooking, coping with other children after school or at bedtimes.

There is no evidence to suggest that any foods should be avoided altogether, but some mothers may observe that certain foods appear to affect their baby's digestion (this may happen with foods that have a short growing season and may be eaten in some quantity, e.g. strawberries).

A mother should drink plenty (but not excessively) so that she is not thirsty. **Do not** recommend an amount by the pint or jug, or the mother may become very uncomfortable, particularly in the first few days following delivery. She should have a drink beside her when breastfeeding, as this is when she is likely to be thirsty. Milk does not have to be taken to produce milk, but it is a good source of protein and calories. It is probably best for a mother to avoid drinking many cups of strong coffee. Caffeine is a drug and may cause a preterm baby to show signs of being restless.

References

1   Neifert MR (1983), Infant problems in breast-feeding. In *Lactation.* Neville MC, Neifert MR. (eds). New York: Plenum Press.
2   Countryman BA (1995) Self-care. In *Breastfeeding and Human Lactation.* Riordan J, Auerbach KG (eds). London: Jones & Bartlett, Ch. 4.
3   Office of Population Censuses and Surveys (1992) *Infant Feeding 1990.* White A, Freeth S, O'Brien M (eds). London: HMSO.
4   World Health Organization (1989) Infant feeding: the physiological basis. *Bulletin* **67** (Suppl.): Ch.2, pp. 21. Geneva: WHO.
5   Lawrence RA (1987) The management of lactation as a physiological process. *Clinics Perinatol Breastfeeding* March **14**: 1–10.

6 Riordan J (1993) Self-care deficits of the breastfeeding mother. In *Breastfeeding and Human Lactation*. Riordan J, Auerbach KG (eds). London: Jones & Bartlett, Ch. 6, pp. 133.

7 Narayan I, Mehta R, Choudhury DK and Jain BK (1991) Sucking on the 'emptied breast': non-nutritive sucking with a difference. *Arch Dis Child*, **66**: 241–244.

8 Budd SC, Erdman SH, Long DM *et al.* (1993) Improved lactation with metoclopramide. *Clin Pediatr*, **32**: 53.

9 Ehrenkranz RA and Ackerman BA (1986) Metoclopramide effect on faltering milk production by mothers of premature infants. *Pediatrics* **78**: 614.

10 Tankeyoon M, Dusitsin N, Chalapati S, Koetsawang S, Saibiang S, Sas M, Gellen JJ, Ayeri O, Gray R, Pinol A and Zegers L (1984) Effects of hormonal contraception on milk volume and infant growth. *Contraception* **30**: 505–522.

11 Valentine CJ, Hurst NM and Schanler RJ (1994) Hindmilk improves weight gain in low-birth-weight infants fed human milk. *J Pediatr Gastroenterol Nutrition* **18**: 474–477.

12 Whitehead RG and Paul AA (1984) Growth charts and the assessment of infant feeding practices in the western world and in developing countries. *Early Hum Dev* **9**: 187–207.

13 Duncan B, Schaefer C, Sibley B and Fonseca NM (1984) Reduced growth velocity in exclusively breast-fed infants. *Am J Dis Child* **138**: 309–313.

14 Dewey KG, Heinig MJ and Nommsen LA (1992) Growth of breast-fed and formula-fed infants from 0 to 18 months: the DARLING study. *Pediatrics* **92**: 1035–1041.

15 Chandra RK (1982) Physical growth of exclusively breastfed infants. *Nutrition Res* **2**: 275.

16 Hitchcock NE and Coy JF (1989) The growth of healthy Australian infants in relation to infant feeding and social group. *Med J Aust* **150**: 306–11.

17 Whitehead RG, Paul AA and Cole TJ (1989) Diet and growth of healthy infants. *J Hum Nutrition Diet* **2**: 73–84.

18 Butte NF, Garza C, Smith EO and Nichols BL (1984) Human milk intake and growth in exclusively breast-fed infants. *J Paediatr* **104**: 187–195.

19 Odent M (1990) The unknown human infant. *J Human Lact* **6**: 6–8.

20 World Health Organization (1989) Infant feeding: the physiological basis. *Bulletin* (Suppl.) **67**: 9–15.

21 Bustemante SA, Jacobs P and Gaines JA. (1983) Body weight, static and dynamic skinfold thickness in small premature infants during the first month of life. *Early Hum Dev* **8**: 217–224.

22 Hormann E (1977) Breastfeeding the adopted baby. *Birth Fam J* **4**: 165.

23 Philips V (1971) Establishment of lactation for the breastfeeding of an adopted baby. *Res Bull Nurs Mothers Assoc Austr* no. 4.

24 Lawrence R (1994) Induced lactation and relactation (including nursing the adopted baby) and cross nursing. In *Breastfeeding: A Guide to the Medical Profession*, 4th edn. London: Mosby, pp. 555–574.

25 Lewis PJ, Devenish C and Kahn C (1980) Controlled trial of meto-

clopramide in the initiation of breastfeeding. *Br J Clin Pharmacol*
9: 217.
26   Kleinman R, Jacobson L, Hormann E *et al.* (1980) Protein values
of milk samples from mothers without biological pregnancies. *J
Pediatr* **67**: 612.
27   Kulski JK, Hartmann PE, Saint WJ *et al.* (1981) Changes in the
milk composition of nonpuerperal women. *Am J Obstet Gynecol*
139: 597.

6 Breastfeeding the vulnerable baby

6.1 Tongue tie

This condition can sometimes interfere with a term baby's ability to breastfeed. If you suspect the septum (frenulum) beneath the baby's tongue is restricting its movement, tell the doctors. In extreme cases the baby's tongue is not rounded at the tip, instead when an attempt is made to protrude it, the tip is 'm' shaped.

In preterm babies, a degree of apparent 'tongue tie' is not uncommon. As the baby grows, the problem usually corrects itself. However, there is a very small percentage of term babies with tongue tie who cannot touch their hard palate with the tip of their tongue or protrude their tongue over their bottom lip. These are the babies who may require minor surgery to release the tie. (This is important not only for successful breastfeeding but also for speech.)

6.2 Cleft lip and/or palate

There is no doubt that breastfeeding presents a challenge to the mother of a baby with either a cleft lip, a cleft palate or both. It requires patience, perseverance and a great deal of commitment from the parents and from the medical and nursing staff, indeed from anyone involved in the care of the mother and baby.

It is very important to support this mother if her decision is to breastfeed. The mother–baby relationship may be enhanced, the baby will receive the benefits of the breastmilk, and one of the potential long-term benefits of breastfeeding a baby with this defect may be the positive effect on the development of the palatal muscles, which are enhanced through the mechanical action of breastfeeding itself. This helps to maintain the patency of the Eustachian tubes, thereby reducing the chances of serious ear problems occurring. These babies have an increased risk of otitis media and continuing ear problems as they grow older.[1]

6.2.1   Cleft lip

As long as the cleft is only in the baby's lip, breastfeeding should be possible. If the mother supports the underside of the breast this may help the baby to maintain the vacuum within his oral cavity.

6.2.2   Cleft palate

Even a small cleft in the palate may cause considerable problems. If the baby cannot maintain a vacuum between his tongue and the palate, he cannot make a teat out of the breast which is a prerequisite for breastfeeding.

Where the cleft is in the baby's hard palate, breastfeeding presents an additional challenge and will certainly require more patience. The area between the hard and soft palate is important in the stimulation of the sucking reflex. This may be diminished in a baby with a lesion in this part of the palate. It helps if the mother's nipple and areola are soft and pliable enough to go easily into the baby's mouth, and the mother has an efficient 'let-down' reflex. It is, therefore, crucial for the mother to be instructed on how to avoid breast engorgement.

The positioning and attachment of the baby is vital to her success in breastfeeding. Different breastfeeding positions should be tried, for it is unlikely that any one conventional position will be appropriate for all of these babies.

Suggested positions may include:

1. The baby in a sitting position, supported across his mother's lap or with the baby supported alongside the mother's side with his legs pointing towards the back of the mother, as in the underarm position (Fig. 6.1(a) and 6.1(b)).
2. The baby on his back with the mother leaning over to let the breast fall directly into his mouth. This position is

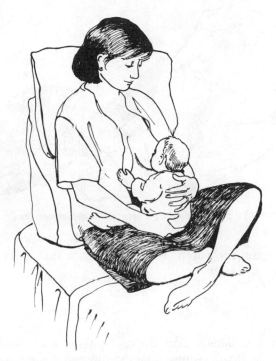

Fig. 6.1(a) *A position for feeding a baby with a cleft abnormality.*

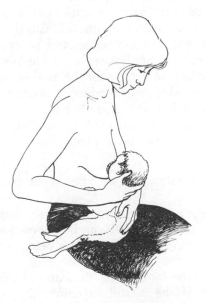

Fig. 6.1(b) *A position for feeding a baby with a cleft abnormality.*

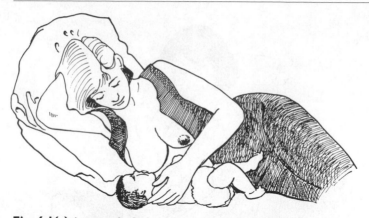

Fig. 6.1(c) *A position for feeding a baby with a cleft abnormality.*

useful for a term baby who has a mature swallow reflex
(Fig. 6.1(c)).

6.2.3   Cleft lip and palate

With a unilateral cleft lip and palate, breastfeeding may be
possible. It will require imagination and flexibility in technique.
All possible feeding positions should be tried, until a suitable
one is found. It may be helpful if the mother is able to insert
her index or little finger just under her breast, so that the breast
tissue enters the baby's mouth and fills the cleft in the lip, thus
creating a seal. The mother should be encouraged to express
regularly to keep her breasts as soft as possible.

It may take several days for the mother and the baby to establish an acceptable breastfeeding technique, and even then, it is
highly probable that the mother will have to supplement her
baby with an additional feeding method until surgical closure
of the lip and palate takes place.

6.2.4   The establishment of breastfeeding

It may help a mother who wishes to breastfeed if the initial
few weeks following birth can be devoted to the establishment
of breastfeeding – without bottles being introduced.

- Once the mother has the baby positioned at the breast,
  even if she is still experimenting with positions, she
  should gently hand express a little milk into the baby's

mouth. This often results in the baby wanting more, whether the baby is preterm or term.

- The baby should be allowed to experiment with suckling at the breast as often as possible. It is not uncommon in these early days for a baby to appear very frustrated at the breast. One important cause may be that the nipple or the teat of a bottle may have gone through the cleft into the naso-pharangeal space, causing the baby difficulty in breathing and swallowing – and causing him to panic and alarming the mother. It may take time to overcome this problem, for to suck effectively the baby has to compress the nipple or teat between two firm surfaces. The nipple or teat may need to be angled in the baby's mouth to achieve this. Breastfeeding may for this reason be an easier option for a baby as the mother's let-down reflex will allow milk to flow with the minimum of compression. It is important for the mother to express after feeding to ensure the breasts receive adequate stimulation.

The mother **must** accept that during this time she **may** have to supplement her baby with an alternative feeding method. This needs to be introduced while the mother is in hospital, partly to assess its suitability, and partly to give the parents time to practice. Bottles **do not** have to be used. A cup, cup and spoon or the nursing supplementer may be used instead.[2,3] If possible, gastric tubes should be removed as soon as possible, as they may hinder a baby's ability to swallow efficiently. Term babies should not require gastric tubes unless there are other problems present at birth.

Even if breastfeeding **is established** in an acceptable way to the mother and her baby, an additional method of feeding may still be necessary until corrective surgery has taken place. Breastfeeding alone may not be able to supply the baby with sufficient volumes of milk to ensure his growth is adequate. This is because the baby is unable to drain the milk sinuses efficiently. It is important therefore, to monitor the baby's growth carefully in the first few days and weeks after breastfeeding is established. Weights should be recorded every 2 days or so. If they are satisfactory, then there is no need to supplement the baby with additional fluids. However, if the weight remains static or weight loss occurs on more than two consecutive occasions, then an additional feeding method will need to be considered. **Do not test weigh** this baby, it will invariably undermine the mother's confidence.

It is important to support the mother in what is a difficult feeding situation, but one in which it is possible for her to succeed. Therefore, any way of maintaining the mother's milk supply, continuing with the breastfeeding so far established and using an acceptable additional feeding method should be encouraged. Time at the breast may be an important positive experience for the baby, particularly if the mother is to establish total breastfeeding once surgery has been performed.

A baby with a bilateral cleft lip and/or palate may also be able to feed from the breast, although this is uncommon. Those who are not able to suckle can still be fed expressed breastmilk by cup,[2,3] or cup and spoon. He can also taste and lick any milk expressed on to the nipple, or take milk directly expressed into his mouth from the breast.

6.2.5   If breastfeeding is not established

If breastfeeding **has not been established** or looks unlikely to become so at the end of a reasonable period of time (for example, 3 weeks), bottle-feeding may be introduced. This does not mean the mother must stop continuing to persevere with breastfeeding as well. Expressed breastmilk can be given by bottle, a variety of teats may need to be experimented with, such as a Habermann teat, a cannon teat, a 'lamb's teat (which is long and soft) or an ordinary teat.

6.2.6   Support groups

The date of any future corrective surgery may also have an influence on the mother's ability to maintain her commitment to breastfeeding and continued expression of breastmilk. If surgery is likely within the first 6 months of life, a baby may well be able to breastfeed afterwards, with the perseverance and patience of the mother. There are several cases where this has occurred, and the mother should contact either the La Leche League or the National Childbirth Trust, both of which have specialized counsellors with direct experience of this situation, and will, therefore, be able to provide the mother with the help and support she will definitely require. Cleft Lip and Palate Association (CLAPA) is the specific support group for parents of babies with a cleft lip and/or palate, and may also be able to give additional help and advice with feeding (the address is given in the Appendix).

6.2.7 General advice

- Make sure this mother knows how to hand express.
- Teach the mother to avoid engorgement.
- Feed the baby in a semi-upright or sitting position, or in any position in which the mother and her baby can satisfactorily complete a feed. The mother laying down with her baby alongside may be a useful position, as the breast can, with gravity, 'fall' far enough into the baby's mouth for the milk to be swallowed, without going into his nose.
- Make sure the baby can suck well, by giving him plenty of practice of sucking on a knuckle or fist, or clean finger rather than on a dummy. This is important so that he becomes used to sucking on an object that is not static in the mouth.
- Encourage the baby to open his mouth widely. The mother can make use of her rooting reflex by gently teasing the baby's cheek or bottom lip with the nipple.
- Always express a small amount of milk on to the nipple prior to attaching the baby at the breast. Direct expression will help a baby to respond to the taste of breastmilk initially and may help the milk to flow more easily.
- Introduce any additional feeding method as early as possible, so the parents have plenty of practice of using it. The cup, cup and spoon, and the nursing supplementer should all be considered for use.
- Breastfeeding may be more successful if a baby's initial hunger is met with her mother's alternative feeding method, and then he is attached to the breast.
- The baby may need 'winding' more frequently than other babies.
- This mother and baby should be discharged when the mother's milk supply is established, the baby's position and attachment at the breast are satisfactory, and the alternative method of feeding being used presents no danger to the baby.

- Ensure the parents are aware of the importance of monitoring their baby's weight and growth regularly.

6.3 Bell's palsy and breastfeeding

If part of a baby's face is temporarily or permanently paralysed, this can cause problems in the commencement and establishment of successful breast- or bottle-feeding.

Bell's palsy is caused by pressure on the seventh cranial nerve. It can arise in three main ways:

1. Most commonly from delivery by forceps. This causes temporary facial paralysis, which usually begins to improve within 24–48 hours, but can last for up to 6 weeks.
2. Pressure *in utero* on the nerve from the pelvic bones. This may cause permanent damage depending upon how long the pressure has existed.
3. Abnormal nerve development causing permanent facial palsy.

The seventh cranial nerve affects movement in the face and the anterior portion of the tongue, possibly interfering with taste. However, the nerves supplying facial sensation and therefore the rooting reflex, movement of the tongue, palate and generally those involved in sucking and breathing are **not** affected.

The main problems are:

- An inability to form a seal with the mouth around the areola or teat.
- An inability to open the mouth as widely as necessary in breastfeeding.

To overcome these problems:

1. Express a little milk on to the nipple at the start of the feed.
2. Position the baby so that the paralysed part of his face is facing away from the breast, therefore, ensuring maximum stimulation for opening the mouth widely.
3. Hold the baby in the underarm position so that his mother has maximum control of his head. Alternatively, the mother may find having the baby laying beside her so that the

breast falls directly into the baby's mouth, a useful position.

4. With the mother's free hand, she can gently hold the baby's chin down to open his mouth wide enough to ensure correct attachment at the breast, making sure the tongue is not in the roof of his mouth (too much pressure on the chin will cause the tongue to be drawn into the back of the baby's mouth).

Encourage the mother initially to express directly into the baby's mouth to encourage him to respond to the taste of the milk. If the problem is temporary, always try the baby at the breast first. If this is unsuccessful, the mother should express her milk and give it to the baby by cup.

A cup may be very useful if the palsy is permanent, although it will also be important to encourage the development of the sucking reflex. A Habermann teat may be useful in this situation.

6.4 Breastfeeding the baby compromised by respiratory and heart problems

Recent evidence suggests that breastfeeding is less stressful to preterm babies than bottle feeding, and that temperature and oxygen levels also remain more stable throughout breastfeeding.[4-6] This can partly be explained by the fact that a baby who breastfeeds can pace his own feeding, in time and quantity, whereas, with bottle feeding it is the person giving the feed who may influence the pace in a number of direct ways (e.g. gently shaking the bottle when the baby stops sucking; making the hole in the teat bigger). A breastfed baby is held very close to his mother's breast with familiar scents, taste and sounds. All of these factors are an advantage for a baby compromised by respiratory or heart problems, and who needs to conserve his energy.

Breastfeeding is not usually a problem for a baby dependent on oxygen, if it is given via nasal cannulae. The positioning and attachment of the baby at the breast to give the nose as much freedom as possible is very important. The underarm position may be the most appropriate to achieve this (Fig. 6.2).

Where oxygen is ambient in the incubator, this also rarely poses a problem, while the baby is out of the incubator, as long

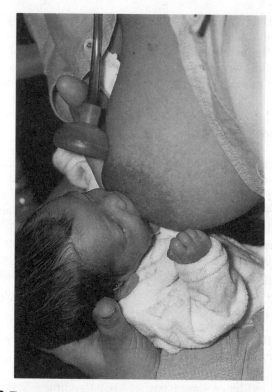

Fig. 6.2 *The position and breast attachment of a baby requiring oxygen therapy. (Photo courtesy of the North Staffs Neonatal Unit and Egnell-Ameda.)*

as oxygen is given via a funnel placed over the mother's shoulder near the baby's nose.

If a baby requires oxygen in a headbox of above 50%, it is better to wait until the oxygen requirement comes down to 30–35% before attempting to breastfeed. An oxygen requirement of 30–35% will not harm an otherwise healthy baby who is held by his mother for a short time with oxygen via a funnel, and at the same time have milk directly expressed into his mouth or the occasional attempt at breastfeeding. It may be necessary to keep this baby attached to an oxygen saturation monitor during his time out of the incubator.

A baby who is tachypnoeic, and/or obviously agitated as well, is best left to rest. However, a baby who has no other symptoms apart from tachypnoea may benefit from being held close to his mother and allowed to feed from the breast if he wishes. The decision to do this must depend upon the baby's condition and the agreement of the doctors.

6.5 Multiple births

Mothers are well able to produce sufficient milk for twins or triplets without supplementation being necessary. For higher order births she may wish to use a formula milk as well, but it depends on the individual mother's milk supply and on her confidence and commitment to breastfeeding her babies herself.

6.6 The preterm baby

Until a preterm baby gives some indication that he is ready to take milk directly from the breast, the mother must express milk so that she can maintain her milk production and supply.

In addition to touching and talking to her baby, the expressing of milk is the singularly most important thing that a mother who wishes to breastfeed can do (particularly for the preterm or sick baby). It is milk unique to that baby and cannot be provided by anyone, other than the mother. It is important that she is aware of this. It is also worth asking mothers, particularly of babies born between 24 and 32 weeks who wish to bottle feed, if they will consider expressing their breastmilk until the baby can tolerate gastric bolus feeds of a formula milk and oral feeds from a bottle.

Whenever possible, the mother should be encouraged to hold her baby. Skin-to-skin contact is ideal.[7] This gives the baby the opportunity to familiarize herself to the mother's scent and the feel of the breast, and encourages bonding in difficult circumstances. It also helps stimulate the mother's milk supply and gives unlimited access to the breast.

Between 32 and 34 weeks and sometimes as early as 30 weeks, the baby will show signs of being more awake, of wanting to suck on anything close by, e.g. his fist, and of not being satisfied by either continuous tube feeds or intermittent feeds via the gastric tube. When this occurs, it is worth encouraging the mother to express directly into the baby's mouth and for cup feeds to be gradually introduced.

It is important that the mother is prepared for the likely sequence of events that her preterm (or sick) baby may go through in order to establish breastfeeding, so that she does not expect too much in the early stages. She should also know how she can avoid problems developing during this period.

The main features of a preterm or sick baby are:

- A weak suck.
- The baby may tire easily.
- A lack of co-ordination in sucking/swallowing/ breathing.
- A preterm baby is immature.

6.6.1   Overcoming the problems

All these problems can be overcome by some or all of the following:

1. At each opportunity when the mother is in the unit, she should, if possible, and depending upon the baby's condition, be able to hold her baby. If milk is hand expressed on to the nipple, the baby should be able to taste it. If the baby wants to try suckling, make sure positioning and attachment are correct so that the baby has no difficulty in taking her milk.
2. The mother or her helper can gently massage the breast towards the nipple, thus encouraging the milk flow. Never try to force the baby to suckle. Suckling **will** eventually occur, but only when the baby is ready – patience and perseverance are the secret!
3. Correct positioning and attachment of the baby is vital to successful breastfeeding, particularly in these early stages. The mother needs to feel competent at positioning so that she can be independent of hospital staff as soon as possible. The underarm position is most suitable for a small baby, where his mouth is small but the nipple appears large. In this position, the mother has control of the baby's head, and can direct the nipple and areola into his mouth more easily. The baby can be encouraged to open his mouth widely by gently brushing her cheek or lips with the mother's nipple, or applying slight pressure on his chin to open his mouth. Too much pressure will be counterproductive as it will cause the tongue to be drawn too far back into his mouth. The mother may find another position more suitable, but as long as she can feed successfully in her chosen position, that is all that matters.
4. A preterm (or sick) baby will initially tire easily. It is useful if the mother starts the milk flow by hand expression before

attaching him to the breast. The baby will organize his sucking pattern differently to a more mature baby. Initially, sucking is for short periods with frequent rests in-between. These rests may last for quite long periods. Gradually, sucking will last for longer periods before resting occurs. If the baby is attached to the breast, encourage his mother to keep him in position and not to move him just because there is a long pause between suckling, or because he appears to be asleep. These very long pauses are completely normal at this stage. If the baby **is** asleep, gently change his position, if he does not stir sufficiently for the feed to continue, then it is best to finish the session and let him rest. If, however, he is still awake but lacks the energy to finish his feed at the breast, he can be given a cup-feed.

5. Frequent attempts to make a preterm baby breastfeed will be counterproductive. It is better to have one concerted effort during the day when the conditions are right, i.e. the baby is awake, hungry and wanting to suckle. At other times, the mother should be encouraged to hold the baby close while being tube fed – but allowing the baby to take milk from the breast in his own time. The baby's readiness to breastfeed becomes obvious from the response shown to his mother, as time continues. Gradually, the mother should be encouraged to be present at more feed times. Before discharge she should be able to stay in the unit for one or two nights if possible, or until she is confident that her baby can feed well. This period is also useful to help wean the mother off the pump, if she has been expressing for a long period of time.

6. For many preterm babies, when they are initially learning to breastfeed, supplementation or replacement of feeds is necessary via a nasal or oral gastric tube or a cup, with either expressed breastmilk or a formula milk. Low birthweight formulae are sometimes prescribed by the doctors, when the baby's weight gain is very slow or static. However, if the mother has an abundant milk supply, suggest she follows the 'hind-milk' regime. The baby should then begin to gain weight more quickly. This is particularly noticeable in the first month of lactation when the protein content of preterm milk is at its highest. If the mother hand expresses her milk, do not divide the milk into separate bottles. Use it all, making certain the bottle is shaken to evenly distribute the fat content before using any milk. If

any formula milk is used, mix it with the mother's own milk, because absorption is likely to be more efficient.

7. Gastric tubes should be removed as quickly as possible as they may delay the co-ordination of the suck and swallow reflex.[8] Cup-feeding is useful because it allows the baby to take what he wants and pace himself. It is also a useful method of supplementing a baby after a breastfeed if this is necessary. It gives the baby the taste of the milk and the added stimulation that this provides, such as exercise of the tongue and jaw muscles, and release of lingual lipases to aid fat digestion. Cup-feeding can be safely used before the baby is able to breastfeed. Parents should be shown how to use this method of feeding.

8. If a baby is taking milk at the breast, providing that it is more than just a few sucks, wait till the baby indicates that he is hungry before supplementing or breastfeeding again. In the initial few feeds, it may be necessary to give a baby a supplementary feed after the breastfeed. In this case, it is better to wait $\frac{1}{2}$–1 hour before giving the tube feed. Small babies often require 2 hourly feeds and, if there are no contraindications, it is better to wait until the next feed is due before any supplemention is given. This depends on the circumstances of each individual baby. The mother should express milk from both of her breasts until the baby is able to drain the breasts efficiently himself.

    Once a baby is taking $\frac{2}{3}$ of his feeds via the breast, he may appear to go for longer or shorter periods than the schedule laid down by a unit on a feed chart. This is normal behaviour for a baby. A preterm baby may well require more frequent feeds until his stomach grows. Gradually he will develop his own routine. It is useful for a baby to receive regular (i.e. 3 hourly) tube feeds overnight so that his mother has more flexibility during the day time.

Weighing the baby every second day is a useful way of assessing his progress once he is able to regulate his own intake and feed times.

6.7 The ventilated baby

A baby who is being ventilated will be able to receive his mother's expressed breastmilk via a transpyloric tube or a gastric tube.

Another way that the mother's milk can also be used is for her baby's mouth care (rather than using sterile water). This will be pleasant for the baby and may additionally stimulate some lingual lipase activity.

A term or preterm ventilated baby who is stable can be held by his mother (or his father), skin-to-skin. This can help to relax the mother and, therefore, encourage her milk flow. It is also very special for either of the parents to be able to touch and comfort their baby, when he is still so fragile and so in need of their special touch and closeness.

6.8 The jaundiced baby

6.8.1 Physiological or idiopathic jaundice

Jaundice is a common condition in babies who are preterm, infected or bruised, following a difficult delivery – particularly after a forceps or after a vacuum extraction. Jaundice is also more common among babies who are breastfed rather than those who are formula fed[9,10] (although this may reflect problems with breastfeeding practice).

The bilirubin level in physiological jaundice usually reaches its peak 3–4 days after delivery.

6.8.2 How to reduce the development of jaundice in the first few days after birth

1. Breastfeeding or the administration of expressed breastmilk (if necessary) should be commenced as soon after birth as possible.
2. Colostrum should be given to a baby because it aids the quick passage of meconium, owing to its laxative effect. It thus prevents the high level of bilirubin contained in meconium being reabsorbed and further increasing the level of jaundice.[11]
3. Demand feeding and good positioning of the baby at the breast, from birth, ensure that the baby receives sufficient colostrum and milk, to either prevent or lessen the development of jaundice.

The following two points are important for term babies with a bilirubin level just below the level requiring phototherapy:

- The baby should be nursed beside his mother.
- The baby should be fed whenever he wants to be.

6.8.3   Pathological or haemolytic jaundice

This kind of jaundice may occur as a result of haemolysis of the baby's blood, owing to an ABO blood incompatability. It may also result from drug therapy given to the baby and on rare occasions result from some disease states of the mother.

The jaundice level peaks at around 24 hours after birth, but jaundice may be present from very soon after delivery in both a term and preterm baby. In very serious cases the baby will require an exchange transfusion. Phototherapy will also be necessary. Breastmilk should be given for his fluid needs and breastfeeding should continue when the baby is sufficiently awake to feed.

6.8.4   Phototherapy and feeding method

When phototherapy is prescribed, additional fluids may be necessary to prevent dehydration. However, for a term or preterm baby who wakes and demands his feed, and breastfeeds well, supplementary fluids will not be required. More frequent feeds may be demanded by the jaundiced baby to counteract any diarrhoea or increased thirst; therefore, any time schedule should be flexible enough to allow true demand feeding – even if this means feeding 1–3 hourly.

Nasal or oral gastric tubes should not be passed unless the baby is very sleepy. Cup-feeding may be a better method of supplementing a baby because a mother can give the cup-feed and hold her baby closely as well.

If a baby is very sleepy when jaundiced, 3 hourly feeds may be necessary, even though he may not be able to breastfeed efficiently. The breast should be offered first of all, if he does not appear interested or is too sleepy, a cup can be offered. If this is also not successful, the feed should be given by a gastric tube, which is then removed after the feed (so that it does not interfere with his potential suckling ability at the next feed).

If a breastfeed is successful, supplementary feeding is not necessary. It can be helpful to the baby if his mother stimulates the milk flow before he begins his feed.

In cases where a jaundiced baby is under phototherapy, and is not waking for feeds or is feeding inadequately, he may require additional fluids via a gastric tube, although a cup may be sufficient. This often applies to babies of 36 weeks or less. Milk should be given as the supplementary or replacement fluid, **not** water or dextrose. The protein in the milk lines the baby's gut, decreasing the reabsorption of unconjugated bilirubin. This does not occur with water or dextrose, and, therefore, increased levels of bilirubin may result. If a mother is unable to express sufficient breastmilk, a formula milk should be used together with her expressed milk, as the two will work more effectively together than formula milk on its own.

The nursing supplementer may help the baby to feed more effectively.

6.8.5   Breastmilk jaundice

The cause of breastmilk jaundice is poorly understood. However, it is the most likely explanation of prolonged jaundice in the newborn breastfed baby (that is jaundice that continues beyond the first week). It is thought that the baby reacts to an unknown substance in the mother's milk. This substance causes some enzyme activity in the baby's liver, which results in a slower breakdown and secretion of bilirubin.

The bilirubin level peaks at around 5–8 days after birth and high levels may persist for several weeks (sometimes as long as 16 weeks), during which time the baby remains jaundiced. It is **not necessary** to stop breastfeeding, and there are no recorded cases of kernicterus with breastmilk jaundice. Occasionally, on medical advice, breastfeeding may be stopped for 12–24 hours (a fall in the serum bilirubin during this period usually confirms the diagnosis). In this case, the mother should express her milk and freeze it until she is able to resume normal breastfeeding. The baby's serum bilirubin level is likely to rise again when breastfeeding is resumed, but generally not to the level it previously reached.[12]

6.9   The unsettled baby

There are numerous reasons for a baby being unsettled at the breast or after a feed. Many, although not connected to breastfeeding, can have a negative effect on its success.

The reasons include:

- The mother's emotional state. If she is tense and anxious.
- The baby may have a dirty nappy or have a sore bottom.
- The baby may be too cold or too hot.
- The baby may have wind or colic.
- The baby may feel insecure and require swaddling.
- The baby may simply want to be cuddled or entertained.
- The baby may have thrush and, therefore, have a sore mouth.
- Too many people may have handled the baby, i.e. the baby may have been held by too many visitors, causing him to be overstimulated.
- The baby may be in a smokey atmosphere if either parent or someone nearby is smoking.

Reasons connected to breastfeeding may include:

- The baby's position and attachment at the breast.
- The let-down reflex may be very strong causing the milk to flow too quickly.
- The mother of a preterm baby may have more milk than the baby requires, causing him to take a lot of fore-milk so that, though full, he still feels hungry. The baby may develop colic as a result.
- Insufficient milk.
- The mother may have eaten something that has affected the taste of her milk (although it appears that the mother's diet, and the subsequent effect it has on the odour and taste of her milk, may influence her baby's readiness to accept certain foods at the time of weaning).[13]
- The mother's menstrual periods may have begun, which can similarly affect the taste of her milk.
- The baby's nose may be blocked by nasal secretions.
- The baby may be squashed against the breast, causing him to panic if she cannot breathe easily.

N.B. Make sure that the baby does not suffer from tongue tie. This will certainly interfere with breastfeeding and cause the baby to be agitated.

Some simple solutions may include:

1. Playing calming music while feeding.
2. Breastfeeding with soft lights in a warm room.
3. Checking the baby's position and attachment are correct at the breast.
4. The baby may be soothed by a warm bath
5. Stroking or massaging the baby with baby oil. This will calm both mother and baby.
6. Using a 'shell' or 'white noise' tape. These are commercial tapes or devices (the shell) which play a continual sound supposed to resemble the womb sounds. They are put close to the baby and are reported to calm him. (A vacuum cleaner and a car engine are supposed to have a similar effect on a baby!) If these tapes are used, they appear to be most effective if played to the baby from birth.
7. A small tape recorder can be put into an incubator. A tape of the mother's and/or father's voice can be played, or a tape of music that was played while the mother was pregnant.
8. Place a used breast pad in the incubator or cot near the baby, so that he can be comforted by the familiar smell.
9. Give the baby 10–15 ml of milk by cup prior to feeding, to calm him.
10. Eliminate any obvious dietary reason for the breastmilk being less palatable to the baby.

Do not time feeds!

6.10   Hypoglycaemia and the breastfed baby

From a practical point of view it is important to **prevent** babies becoming hypoglycaemic, that is having a low blood sugar level, at birth or later on. This is important in view of concern raised about the relationship between neonatal hypoglycaemia and neurological damage.[14]

6.10.1   Which babies are at risk?

An assessment of a baby can be made at birth to see whether he falls into a high- or low-risk category of becoming hypoglycaemic. The following criteria can be used to make this assessment.

High-risk factors

- The baby is less than 36 completed weeks gestation at birth.
- The baby is less than 2.5 kg at birth.
- The baby is cold at or after the birth.

(The mother experienced a long and difficult labour; prolonged rupture of membranes, thus predisposing her baby to infection. The mother is a poorly controlled diabetic, with unstable blood sugars.)[15]

Low-risk factors

- The baby is more than 36 completed weeks gestation at birth.
- The baby is between 2.5 and 4.5 kg at birth.
- The baby has Apgar scores of 5 or more at 1 minute, at birth.

(The mother is healthy, the labour and delivery were uncomplicated, with no prolonged rupture of membranes. She is a well-controlled diabetic, with stable blood glucose levels.)

The baby should have a normal temperature, colour, breathing pattern and muscle tone.

6.10.2   Breastfeeding and the low-risk baby

There is little national concensus on the normal lower limit of the blood sugar level, either for the term or preterm baby. According to Hawdon *et al.*,[16] neonatal hypoglycaemia is defined as a blood sugar level of below 2.6 mmol/l, though other definitions may be lower than this.[17] It is known, however, that term breastfed babies, who are also of an appropriate weight for their gestational age, have a lower blood sugar in the first week of life compared to formula-fed babies. Therefore, in the first 3 days, a breastfed baby may have blood sugar levels below 2.6 mmol/l.[16] The response of a **term, healthy baby** to a low blood sugar is to make use of the body's alternative sources of fuel, such as ketone bodies from fatty acids released from the baby's fat stores. Therefore, unless the baby shows symptoms of hypoglycaemia (these include jitteriness, apnoea, an abnormal cry, poor feeding, tremor, hypertonia and, if extreme, convulsions), there is no real necessity to either test the blood sugar level or interfere with his routine of breastfeeding in the first few days of life. Research indicates that it is uncommon for a term baby to have a low blood sugar after the third post-natal day.[16]

To help prevent hypoglycaemia from developing a baby needs to be fed **early and on 'demand'**, ensuring that the baby is well attached and positioned, from birth. Some newborn babies, however, may sleep for long periods after birth and between initial feeds. This may result in blood sugar levels **below 2.6 mmol/l**, but, as long as the babies are asymptomatic and their temperature, colour, breathing pattern and muscle tone are all normal, they are unlikely to require any extra feeding. How long a term, healthy baby is left to sleep depends to a large extent upon local policy.

6.10.3 Breastfeeding and the high-risk baby

The preterm, low birthweight and sick baby are all in high-risk categories of potentially developing hypoglycaemia. The preterm and low birthweight babies (i.e. small and/or light for gestational age) do not have the extra fat stores of the term healthy baby to compensate for a low blood sugar. Therefore, maintenance of their blood sugar level is critical.

Where gastric or oral feeds are possible, they should be commenced **early and be given regularly**. It is suggested that, where preterm and low birthweight babies have regular feeds of 120 ml/kg/day, persistent hypoglycaemia is unlikely to occur and that enteral feeding itself may help to stimulate ketone body production.[16] Breastfeeding should be encouraged whenever possible with the high-risk babies, but they may need to be regularly monitored – not only to ensure they remain asymptomatic but also initially to ensure that they maintain a stable blood sugar level.

If the baby **cannot** breastfeed at this time, he should be given any colostrum the mother can express, together with any artificial formula or banked human milk considered necessary. This can be given by cup or gastric tube. The high-risk baby should initially be given feeds regularly, i.e. 2–3 hourly according to the advice of the paediatrician, with breastfeeds offered before any other method of feeding is used if this is possible. The baby's temperature, colour, breathing pattern and muscle tone should be assessed at each feed, and blood sugar level checked at the same time.

If after a prescribed period of time the blood sugar level has remained above 2.6 mmol/l (or whatever is considered appropriate according to local policies), then further testing can be discontinued. It is important, however, to continue to give the baby regular feeds, gradually reducing them from 2–3 hourly to 4 hourly, and to demand feeding. If the blood sugar level is considered to remain low, the baby should be assessed by the paediatrician. The mother should continue to express her colostrum and milk until her baby can breastfeed efficiently. The mother should also offer her breast whenever the baby is fed.

Intravenous glucose may be necessary if oral or gastric feeding is not tolerated or not initially possible.

6.11 Bowels and the breastfed baby

Colostrum has a mild but nevertheless important laxative effect, which encourages the passage of meconium.[11] If it is given early and regularly to a baby, it will help prevent the development of jaundice, by preventing reabsorption of bilirubin from the meconium.

6.11.1 Colour and consistency

Meconium is the very dark brown/black/greeny, thick and tarry stool, which is present from birth. After 2 or 3 days, a 'changing stool' should be passed, which is brown in colour. This indicates that the baby is getting his mother's milk. This stool may be quite loose. Thereafter, the stool should be mustard yellow in colour, soft to loose in consistency with a slightly curdled appearance.

Any change in consistency or colour is likely to indicate a change in the mother's diet.

6.11.2 Warning signs

- A term baby passing meconium at 4–5 days is clearly not getting enough milk.

- A changing stool at 4–5 days similarly may indicate a need to examine the feeding technique (such as, positioning and attachment, any restriction on frequency of feeds, the length of time the baby spends at the breast).
- A green stool may indicate the baby is getting insufficient milk.

6.11.3   Frequency of bowel actions

Breastfed babies have little waste to excrete; therefore, they do not necessarily have a regular bowel pattern. Some babies may only pass two or three stools in a week. As long as the baby is otherwise healthy, gaining weight satisfactorily and is passing urine, there is no need to worry.

6.12   Thrush and breastfeeding

If a mother has persistently sore/inflamed nipples and areola, at and between feeding times, and/or if a baby is unwilling to suck at the breast, always check the baby's mouth (and nappy area) for a thrush infection. Thrush appears as either a white-coated tongue, or as curd-like white patches inside his mouth and cheeks, which cannot be wiped away. In this case, both mother and baby need to be treated with an anti-fungal preparation, such as Nystatin or Daktarin.

When a baby is being treated with antibiotics, thrush is always a possibility. Be very vigilant in carrying out anti-thrush treatment as prescribed, using oral preparations before breastfeeding to prevent spread to the mother. (A thrush infection in the mother may present as a persistant breast pain. It may require treatment with a systemic anti-fungal preparation.)

6.13   HIV and breastfeeding

A mother who is known to be HIV-antibody positive, or who is at a high risk of contracting the disease is advised to avoid breastfeeding.[18] However, because heat pasteurization of expressed breastmilk at 62.5°C for 30 minutes kills the HIV virus,[19] the mother's milk could in some circumstances be used to feed **her own** baby.

If a mother decides that she wants to provide her own milk for her baby, hand expression would be the best method of method of milk removal. If a pump is used, the mother should have it for her own exclusive use, for the duration of her lactation.

References

1 Paradise J, Elster B and Tan L (1994) Evidence in infants with cleft palate that breast milk protects against otitis media. *Pediatrics* **94**: 853–860.

2 Lang S, Lawrence CJ and L'E Orme R (1994) Cup feeding: an alternative method of infant feeding. *Arch Child Dis* **71**: 365–369.

3 Lang S (1994) Cup-feeding: an alternative method. *Midwives Chronicle* **107**: 171–176.

4 Meier P (1988) Bottle- and breast-feeding: effects on transcutaneous oxygen pressure and temperature in preterm infants. *Nursing Res* **37**: 36–40.

5 Meier P and Pugh E (1985) Breast-feeding behaviour of small preterm infants. *Am J Mat Child Nurs* **10**: 396–401.

6 Meier P and Anderson GC (1987) Responses of small preterm infants to bottle and breast feeding. *Am J Mat Child Nurs* **12**: 97–105.

7 Whitelaw A, Heisterkamp G, Sleath K *et al.* (1988) Skin to skin contact for very low birthweight infants and their mothers. *Arch Dis Child* **63**: 1377–1381.

8 Kelnar JH and Harvey D (1987) Nutrition. In *The Sick Newborn Baby*, 2nd edn. Kelnar JH and Harvey D (eds). London: Baillère Tindall, pp. 134–159.

9 Salariya EM and Robertson CM (1993) Relationship between baby feeding types and patterns and gut transit time of meconium and the incidence of neonatal jaundice. *Midwifery* **9**: 235–242.

10 Schneider AP (1986) Breastmilk and jaundice in the newborn – a real entity. *JAMA* **225**: 3270–3274.

11 De Carvalho M, Klaus MH and Merkatz RB (1982) Frequency of breast-feeding and serum bilirubin. *Am J Dis Child* **136**: 737–738.

12 Auerbach KG and Gartner LM (1987) Breastfeeding and human milk: their association with jaundice in the neonate. *Clin Perinatol* **14**: 89–107.

13 Sullivan SA and Birch LL (1994) Infant dietary experience and acceptance of solid foods. *Pediatrics* **2**: 271–277.

14 Koh THHG, Aynsley-Green A and Tarbit M (1988) Neuronal dysfunction during hypoglycaemia. *Arch Dis Child* **63**: 1353–1358.

15 Hawdon JM, Ward-Platt MP and Aynsley-Green A (1993) Neonatal hypoglycaemia – blood glucose monitoring and baby feeding. *Midwifery* **9**: 3–6.

16 Hawdon JM, Ward-Platt MP and Aynsley-Green A (1992) Patterns of metabolic adaption in term and preterm infants in the first postnatal week. *Arch Dis Child* **67**: 357–365.

17 Crase BL (1995) Hypoglycaemia and the breastfed newborn (editorial). *Breastfeeding Abstracts* **15**: 11–12.

18 Royal College of Midwives (1991) Notes on less common problems. In *Successful Breastfeeding*, 2nd edn. London: Churchill Livingstone, pp. 69–74.

19. McDougal JS (1990) Pasteurisation of human breast milk and its effect on HIV infectivity. Presentation at the *Annual Meeting of the Human Milk Banking Association of North America*, Lexington, KY, 15 October.

7 Alternative methods of feeding and breastfeeding

7.1 Alternative and supplementary methods of feeding

Alternative and supplementary methods of feeding are gastric and transpyloric tubes, direct expression, cup-feeding, nursing supplementer, syringes and droppers, finger 'assessment' of feeding and bottle feeding.

In certain circumstances, an aid or alternative to breastfeeding may be required, for example, if a mother is a patient in another hospital or ill at the time of her baby's admission to a neonatal or paediatric unit, or a baby is preterm or sick and unable to take a full breastfeed.

The following guidelines describe various options available to the mother and to those who support her. Finger 'assessment' of feeding is included, not because it is an alternative method of feeding but because it can be a useful diagnostic method of assessing a baby's ability to suck and swallow effectively.

7.2 Gastric and transpyloric tubes

7.2.1 Transpyloric tubes

A transpyloric tube is most commonly used when a baby is ventilated to reduce the risk of aspiration. The tube passes into the jejunum and sometimes beyond. However, this method of feeding has a number of drawbacks. It delivers the breastmilk directly into the gut, by-passing the baby's mouth and the stomach, thus reducing important areas of digestion. Depending upon where in the baby's gut the tube is situated, nutrient absorption may also be reduced, leading to an unsatisfactory weight gain.[1] Feeds administered by this route are given continuously.

Expressed breastmilk is the preferred milk type for transpyloric tube-feeding because it is less of an irritant to the gut and therefore, less likely to cause necrotizing enterocolitis.

7.2.2 Gastric tubes

Gastric tubes (Fig. 7.1) are commonly used until a baby is able to sustain his own nutritional requirements, either by breast- or bottle-feeding, or an alternative method of feeding.

Gastric feeding-tubes should not be used for longer than they are absolutely necessary. It has been shown that milk lipids can stick to the sides of the tubes, thus reducing the amount of fat (and calories) available to the baby.[2] It is also suggested that gastric tubes delay the co-ordination of sucking and swallowing.[3]

7.2.3 Continuous and 1–2 hourly bolus tube-feeding

If a baby has a dental plate/obdurator in place, it may be designed to have an oral gastric tube fitted into it. Otherwise a nasal gastric tube securely positioned at the nose or an oral gastric tube securely positioned at the side of the baby's mouth and cheek are used. Continuous gastric tube feeds may be given initially until gastric tolerance and emptying are established. It is then usual for 1 hourly bolus feeds to be commenced, with the feeds gradually becoming less frequent as the baby is able to tolerate larger volumes.

Continuous pump feeds

This is a convenient way to administer expressed breastmilk.

- The syringe should be positioned so that the nozzle is uppermost, thereby ensuring delivery of the richer milk first (which contains increased calories).
- To make certain the milk is kept as fresh as possible, and to reduce the chance of bacterial growth, put only 4

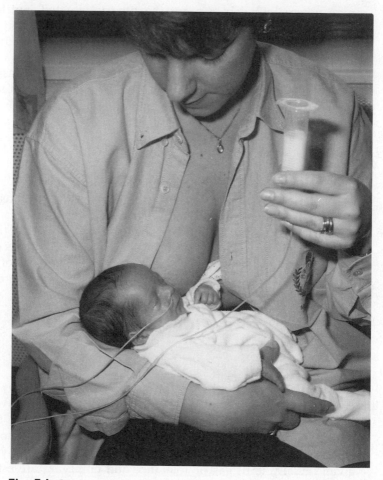

Fig. 7.1 *Gastric tube-feeding. (Photo courtesy of the North Staffs Neonatal Unit and Egnell-Ameda.)*

hours' worth of milk in the syringe at a time, and keep the remainder refrigerated or frozen until required.

1–2 hourly bolus tube-feeding

If the baby is awake at the time of bolus feeds given by gastric tube, a dummy may be used to give him an opportunity to 'suck'. If the mother is present when these 1–2 hourly bolus milk feeds are given, encourage the mother to express some breastmilk on to her nipple for the baby to taste at the same time. Position the baby so that if he shows signs of wanting to suckle, he can easily be attached to the breast. It is preferable for the baby to get his experience of sucking at the breast rather than on a dummy.

7.2.4 Breastfeeding and gastric tubes

Breastfeeding can be commenced with a gastric tube in place. The positioning of the baby is very important. If the baby has a dental plate, the underarm position may be the most practical. The mother should be aware that, because of the plate (unless she has a very protractile nipple or a very supple areola), the baby may not be able to get much areola into his mouth and may not have a very effective suck until the plate is removed. However, one can be proven **wrong**, and some very determined babies will suck very strongly with a plate in position! Gently expressing milk straight into the baby's mouth can be very useful in this situation.

A dental plate with a gastric tube fitted into it should be removed as soon as the plate is no longer clinically required, so that the baby's palate is stimulated when he is attached to the breast.

Dental plates, with a wire loop attached at the back of the plate to encourage swallowing, should be removed at the time of feeding, but left in place between feeds.

Nasal gastric tubes **should be avoided** in the following situations:

- Nasal prong oxygen (reducing the space for a further nasal tube).
- Breathing difficulties.
- Cleft palate.

Breastfeeding with a nasal gastric tube in place is easier than with an oral gastric tube. However, the tube is in the nose and, therefore, cuts down some of the baby's nasal space and breathing capacity. It is important to make sure, in positioning and attachment, that the baby's nose is left as free as possible. The baby should be positioned so that the tube-free nostril is facing away from the nipple. Oral gastric tubes should be secured at the side of the mouth and cheek, to ensure free tongue movement (rather than over the bottom lip and secured on the chin, which considerably restricts movement of the tongue) (Figs 7.2 and 7.3).

The following points are **important** to consider when a baby has a gastric tube in place and the mother wishes to breastfeed her baby.

Continuous gastric tube feeds

Stop the pump during any attempt at breastfeeding.

1–2 hourly bolus gastric tube feeds

1. Put the baby to the breast **before** the next gastric feed is due.
2. On the initial occasion at the breast, direct expression will help a baby to become accustomed to the taste and smell of the milk, and attachment is made much simpler.
3. If a baby is unable to take a feed, or only takes a little, give the bolus via the tube while he is near or attached to the breast. Either the mother can gently express some milk for her baby to taste, or she can hold him close to the breast during the feed.
4. If a baby is able to take some good sucks from the breast, slightly **delay** the next bolus feed.
5. If the mother and hospital staff are happy that her baby has suckled well, DELAY the bolus feed for at least 1 hour or until the baby wants to feed again (whichever is sooner). While the baby is on 1 or 2 hourly feeds, waiting will not

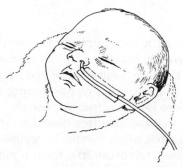

Fig. 7.2 *Securing a nasal gastric tube*

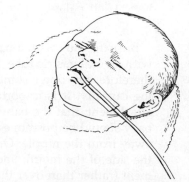

Fig. 7.3 *Securing an oral gastric tube.*

harm a healthy, preterm baby and will 'boost' the mother's confidence enormously.

6. If a tube is due to be changed, give the mother and her baby the opportunity to breastfeed without the tube in place.

7. If possible, begin to introduce a cup once a baby is on 2 hourly intermittent gastric tubes. Quite apart from the tactile experience, it is not stressful, and the baby can taste the milk and stimulate his tongue muscles and digestive juices, and generally enjoy his feed!

3 hourly bolus gastric tube feeds

Initially, these feeds may be via a nasal gastric tube left in place between feeds. Intermittent oral gastric tubes should be used as soon as possible so that the baby can also develop his ability to suck and swallow without any tubes in place. Breastfeeding should be attempted whenever possible, according to the baby's condition.

Cup-feeding should be considered instead of tube feeding whenever possible, but should not be used instead of breastfeeding.

When formula milk has to be used

There are several situations where baby formula milk has to be used with expressed breastmilk. This is inevitable when a mother is not producing sufficient milk for her baby's needs and where low-birthweight formulae are prescribed by the doctors.

Human milk itself contains two lipases. One of these, the bile salt-stimulated lipase (BSSL) possibly aids improved fat absorption when a mixture of formula milk and the mother's own milk is given to a baby.[5] Therefore, any formula milk used should be mixed with a quantity of expressed breast milk, even if this a very small portion of the total amount. Quite apart from the benefits to the baby, it helps the mother to feel her milk remains an important factor in her baby's progress.

7.3 Direct expression of breastmilk

Hand expression of breastmilk directly into the baby's mouth may be commenced whenever he shows signs of wanting to suckle or is held next to his mother's breast (Fig. 7.4) – as long as the baby is not being ventilated at the time. However, it will not harm a baby as nasal continuous positive airway pressure (CPAP) if he wants to lick milk from the breast whilst being held. Some babies on nasal CPAP are even able to suckle without any problem, although this should only be attempted if the baby shows that he is ready, i.e. he 'roots' or begins to suck on the nipple.

Babies as young as 30 weeks (and sometimes earlier) can safely cope with a few drops of their mother's milk in this way. Indeed, breastmilk, unlike formula milk, is not considered to be an irritant to the pulmonary tree if a little is aspirated.[6] However, this eventuality should be avoided.

Direct expressing is useful for a baby who is about to be introduced to breastfeeding. It is a particularly useful technique for a baby who is preterm, weak or sick because it requires little effort. It is also useful for a baby who initially fights at the breast or who is reluctant to suck. It gives the baby the taste of the milk, thereby stimulating the release of oral juices containing enzymes, which aid digestion. It also stimulates the movement of the jaw muscles and tongue, and encourages co-ordination of the suck and swallow reflex. There is nearly always a positive response in the baby.

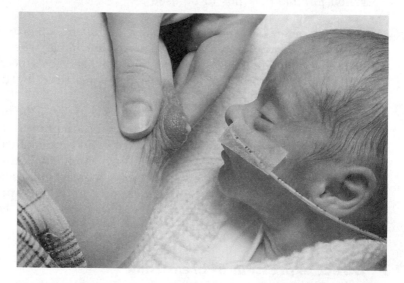

Fig. 7.4 *The direct expression of breastmilk. (Photo courtesy of the North Staffs Neonatal Unit and Egnell-Ameda.)*

It is imperative, if this technique is used, that the mother knows how to hand express correctly.

7.4   Cup-feeding

The main use of cup-feeding (Fig. 7.5) is to provide an alternative method of feeding for a preterm or term baby who is to be breastfed, or is already breastfeeding, and for whom a gastric tube may be temporarily or permanently inappropriate, or unnecessary.[7-9] However, it also provides a satisfactory method of feeding babies with a cleft lip and/or palate. It should also be tried in situations where breast- or bottle-feeding is initially unsuccessful, as in some babies who are unable to co-ordinate their suck, swallow and breathing reflexes in the first few months of life, and therefore, cannot be fed at the breast or from a bottle.

7.4.1   General reasons for using a cup

- To provide a positive oral experience for a baby.
- To provide an alternative method of feeding, when a mother is not available to breastfeed her baby.

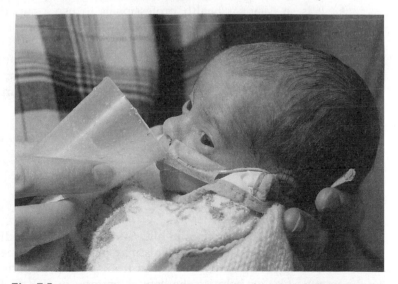

Fig. 7.5 *A preterm baby cup-feeding. (Photo courtesy of the North Staffs Neonatal Unit and Egnell-Ameda.)*

- To avoid any possibility of a baby having problems in breastfeeding as a result of being introduced to different sucking techniques.
- To reduce the need for nasal and oral gastric tubes.

Advantages of cup-feeding

- The baby paces his own intake in time and quantity.
- Little energy is used.
- It stimulates the development of the suck and swallow reflexes, co-ordination is also encouraged.
- Saliva and lingual lipases are stimulated, leading to a more efficient digestion of breastmilk.[10,11]
- Less fat is lost with a cup than via gastric tubes.
- Good eye contact is encouraged between the baby and the person giving the feed.
- The baby has to be held closely and securely for the feed.
- It is a **very easy** method of feeding.

Disadvantages of cup-feeding

- Term babies tend to dribble!
- Term healthy babies can become addicted to the cup if they cannot go to the breast regularly.
- It is **so** easy for health professionals to use a cup that occasionally it is used when it may be more appropriate to try the baby at the mother's breast.
- If the cup is held too tightly in contact with the baby's lips or gums, the skin can be blistered or broken. This is **not** common, but can occur if the cup has a sharp rim or is not held in a relaxed manner.

N.B. A cup must not replace breastfeeding without very good reason.

7.4.2   When and how to use a cup

A cup should be used when an alternative method of feeding to the gastric tube is required. This may be because the baby is not able to feed from the breast or from a bottle (if he is to be formula fed), or because the baby is preterm or sick, or the mother is not present on the unit to breastfeed.

The preterm baby

A cup can be safely used to feed a healthy, preterm baby from approximately 30 weeks gestation, or when a baby shows signs that he is becoming more active orally. It is possible for a baby to cup-feed **before** he is able to breastfeed efficiently. However, it should **never** be used instead of a breastfeed, i.e. where the baby is able to satisfy all, or part of his nutritional needs from the breast. Ideally cup-feeding and learning to breastfeed should take place at the same time.

A cup may be appropriate when

- A preterm baby is wide awake and restless at feed times.
- The baby is showing signs of wanting to suck, e.g. sucking on his fist.
- The baby is not satisfied by tube feeds and is restless after the feed.
- The baby is not yet able to feed directly from the breast, or has only enough energy to satisfy part of his total nutritional needs at the breast.

The majority of preterm babies receive their milk via nasal or oral gastric tubes. Cup-feeding may be commenced when 2–3 hourly bolus tube feeds are introduced or established. It is not usually appropriate whilst continuous or 1 hourly bolus feeds are required or where there is evidence that the baby is not absorbing his milk feeds.

There is some evidence to suggest gastric tubes can delay the development of the suck and swallow co-ordination in babies.[3] This is a particularly important factor to consider when cup-feeding preterm babies, for one of its purposes is to encourage the development of these reflexes and their co-ordination. It is vital, therefore, that gastric tubes are removed as soon as possible. However, it must be left to the discretion of the carer whether it is possible or appropriate to remove a gastric tube prior to a cup-feed.

A preterm baby having only one or two feeds a day by any alternative method should have the tube left in place. When three or more feeds are given by a method other than a gastric tube the tube should be removed, initially to see how well the baby does without it. The tube may have to be replaced and it is important for parents to be aware of this possibility. At this stage, an intermittent oral tube may be more appropriate.

When the baby is initially being introduced to the breast and having the occasional cup-feeds as well, it may be a useful compromise to give the baby gastric tube feeds overnight and alternate the breast with cup during the day. If supplementary feeds are still required, these can be given **after** the breastfeed by cup. Otherwise the cup should be used instead of the tube when the baby is able to go to the breast successfully on three or more occasions a day. The gastric tube should be removed at this time, but should be replaced if there is any concern over the baby's weight gain.

When preterm babies cup-feed, they are often observed to 'lap', by protruding their tongue and taking an amount of milk on their tongue, thus they are also learning to cope with small boluses of milk in their mouths. As they mature, they begin to 'sip' the milk. It is normal for a range of facial expressions to be seen after stimulation of the lips with the cup. At no time should cup-feeding cause distress to a baby. If it does, it may be that either the baby is being held in an inappropriate position, e.g. semi-reclining position, or the cup is placed too far forward on the upper lip or pressing on the lower lip or gums. It may also indicate that milk is being tipped into the baby's mouth, causing him to panic.

The term baby

Cup-feeding is inappropriate for a term healthy baby who can maintain his nutritive needs at the breast. It may, however, be useful if the mother has had a Caesarian section or is ill following delivery, or if the baby requires any oral drugs. Very occasionally cup-feeding may also help a term baby who has become used to a bottle teat or dummy and is having difficulty correctly attaching to the breast. In this case, when repeated attempts to attach this baby to the breast have failed and the mother feels a bottle is her only choice, a cup can be used for up to 24 hours (using the mother's expressed breastmilk) before trying to re-establish breastfeeding again. It may help to use a position for breastfeeding which is different to the one used previously. Special attention should be paid to the attachment of the baby. If a gastric tube has been used to feed a term baby on a neonatal or paediatric unit, then progression to cup-feeding should follow the same guidelines as for the preterm baby. Some term babies refuse cup-feeding altogether, while other term babies who become used to cup-feeding may become addicted to a cup and have to be weaned from it. Where a cup is used with a term healthy or sick baby, it is important to let the baby feed as often as possible at the breast to avoid this.

7.4.3   The baby with special requirements

Much of what has already been written applies in the situation of a baby with special requirements. Cup-feeding in the following two situations is particularly useful.

The baby with a cleft lip and/or cleft palate

Cup-feeding should be used if there is a possibility that the baby will be able to breastfeed. It can be used in the period during which establishment of breastfeeding is taking place. It is helpful to give an initial small amount by cup so that the baby is less frustrated initially at the breast. The direct expression of breastmilk is also very important in establishing breastfeeding with these babies. A cup can be used for a unilateral and bilateral cleft lip and palate.

The baby who cannot suck effectively

Cup-feeding has a particularly important role in the feeding of babies unable to feed from either the breast or a bottle. After it has been established that the baby's ability to suck from the nipple or teat is compromised, but the baby is able to swallow without difficulty, try cup-feeding, particularly if the only alternative is to remain on gastric tube feeds for a prolonged period of time (e.g. several weeks or months).

The baby 'laps' or 'sips' the milk initially from a cup, an action which is frequently possible with babies who have neurological problems. The baby's ability to suck may develop slowly and gradually along with his ability to co-ordinate his suck, swallow and breathing reflexes. This may take from a few days to several months. Cup-feeding encourages the co-ordinated movement of the tongue and muscles of the mouth, while also allowing the baby to enjoy his feeds. This may be very important in the future of this baby. The early feeding experiences are often of great importance, particularly if the child can associate feeding with pleasant experiences. Passing gastric tubes over long periods can be a nerve-racking experience for nursing staff, parents and for the child. Parents can safely cup-feed a baby at home.

If the mother wishes to breastfeed her baby, encourage skin-to-skin contact, the expression of milk on to her nipples or into her baby's mouth which will help to stimulate his tongue movement. Gently stroking the baby's lips will also help to stimulate him to open his mouth. A mother may find these simple strategies more rewarding than giving her baby a dummy because although the baby may be able to suck on a dummy, the technique he adopts may not be correct for successful nutritive sucking at the breast. If it is necessary to assess the baby's sucking ability, it is preferable to use a clean finger. As time passes, the baby may be able to suck efficiently, not only on a dummy, but may also be able to breast- or bottle-feed successfully. Patience and perseverance are certainly needed.

7.4.4   How much should the baby take?

This will depend upon a number of factors:

1. Initially a preterm baby may only take a small amount from the cup, maybe 5–10 ml. This is particularly the case for an immature baby. It is worth giving him the opportunity of cup-feeding at least once a day. He should then be given the rest of his feed via the gastric tube. The baby's response is usually very positive.
2. Once the baby is taking two or more cup-feeds a day, unless a very small amount has been taken and there is good reason, **do not top him up** – wait until the baby wants more milk, or the next feed. A baby at any gestation may want very little milk at one feed and a lot at the next. It is the 24 hour total that is important.
3. However, if the baby has taken at least half of his requirement at a particular feed it is preferable to wait until he next wants more milk. If the baby is not yet waking to demand his feeds and is having 2 hourly feeds, wait till the next feed is due. If he is on 3 hourly feeds, also wait until the next feed is due (if this is possible) or for at least 1 hour before 'topping up', particularly if a gastric tube has to be passed.
4. In the case of a baby who is capable of breastfeeding but not yet able to satisfy all his needs from the breast, allow

him to have more milk from a cup after the feed. The amount he takes should not be regulated, unless the baby is fluid restricted or the breastfeed was very short!

5.   If a preterm (or term) baby initially 'fights' at the breast and direct expression does not help, give a small amount of milk by cup before the breastfeed continues, to settle him.

7.4.5   Method of cup-feeding

The method of cup-feeding is the same for any baby regardless of gestation.

What to use in hospital

A 60 ml medicine measure makes an ideal cup, as long as the rim is not too sharp. These can easily be sent to the hospital's sterilizing unit. Cups with lids and with a rounded rim are available, the advantage of these is that a mother can express milk straight into the cup, which can then either be put into a freezer or into a refrigerator.

What to use at home

An egg cup can be used as long as it has a reasonably thin, rounded rim. It should be made in one piece so that bacteria cannot contaminate the milk from any joins. Also useful for use as a cup is the hard plastic cover for a teat in a bottle set, as long as the rim is rounded and smooth. Some commercially available hand-pump sets may include cups rather than bottles.

Method for feeding

1.   Wrap the baby securely, to prevent his hands knocking the cup. Use a terry nappy placed under his chin. (This can be weighed both prior to, and after the feed, if necessary – for dribble factor!)
2.   Support the baby in an upright sitting position (Fig. 7.6).
3.   If possible have the cup at least half full for the beginning of the feed. (This is particularly helpful for the person learning the technique, so that milk is not poured into the baby's mouth.)
4.   The cup should be tipped so the milk is just touching

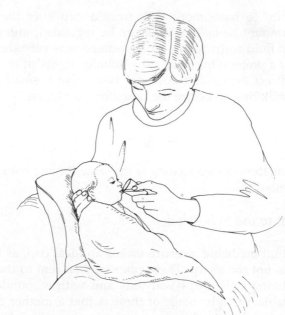

Fig. 7.6 *The position to hold a baby for cup-feeding.*

the baby's lips. It should **not** be poured into the baby's mouth.

5.   Direct the rim of the cup towards the corners of the upper lip and gums, with it gently touching/resting on the baby's lower lip. Do not apply pressure to the lower lip.
6.   Leave the cup in the correct position during the feed. Do not keep removing it when the baby stops drinking. It is important to let the baby pace his own intake in his own time.

Type of milk to use

Expressed breastmilk is the ideal milk to use. However, formula milk can also be given by cup.

N.B. Always shake the bottle containing expressed milk to ensure a more even distribution of the milk fat.

7.5   The nursing supplementer

This is a very useful device, which can be used in a variety of different situations (see Fig. 7.7). Essentially it enables a mother

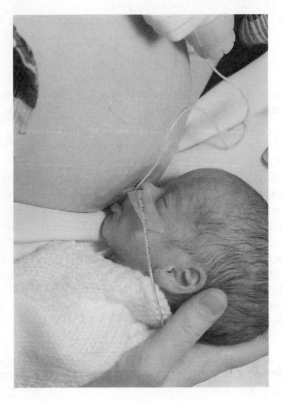

Fig. 7.7 *The nursing supplementer. (Photo courtesy of the North Staffs Neonatal Unit and Egnell-Ameda.)*

and her baby to breastfeed successfully in circumstances which may seem unpromising.

It should be considered in the following situations:

1. Affecting the mother:

   - A genuine low milk production.
   - Persistent insufficient milk supply.
   - Breast surgery.
   - Relactation (after established breast feeding, or to initiate lactation in the case of adoption).

2. Affecting the baby:

   - A weak suck, owing to prematurity.
   - A weak suck, owing to neurological damage.
   - A baby with a weak suck, owing to a chromosomal abnormality, i.e. Down's syndrome.

- A cross baby who will not attach on to the breast.

7.5.1 Method

It is important to attach the nursing supplementer to the breast correctly.

1. Fill the container with the required amount of milk.
2. Make sure the lid is on securely.
3. Hang the container around the neck, so that it hangs between the breasts in a position level with the nipples or just above.
4. Attach the tubes to the nipples. Each tube should be secured in a position on the top of the breasts, with the tip of each tube very slightly protruding over the end of each nipple. The tape used to secure the tubes should be placed above the areola.
5. Position the baby and attach to the breast in the normal way.

If the supplementer has a valve system it may be necessary to release the valve at this point so that the milk flows freely as the baby suckles.

It is important to choose the correct size tubing for the baby – some designs come with a variety of different tube sizes, from the equivalent of a 0.4 to a 0.8 gauge feeding tube. Initially it is useful to begin with the largest size. If the baby is to be breastfed in the future without the supplementer, then the narrower tubes can be gradually introduced, so that less milk is obtained from the supplementer, and more is taken from the mother.

It is also important to control the milk flow as appropriate. As the baby's suck grows stronger and/or the mother's milk flow increases, so the milk flow from the nursing supplementer should be lessened. Some models have a series of notches in the lid into which the tube can be fixed. These are used to slow or reduce the milk flow or completely stop it.

The position of the tubes at the nipple may also need to be adjusted as the need for the nursing supplementer lessens, as some babies can and do become addicted to the tube! The tube can gradually be moved around the areola until it is on the underside, it can then be withdrawn completely. Alternatively the tube can be attached further up the breast until it is no longer in the baby's mouth.

The baby is able to take what he wants from the mother, in addition to the milk in the nursing supplementer. It is important not to supplement the baby after the feed on the evidence of what has been taken from the visible milk supply. It is better to rely on how the mother feels:

- Do her breasts feel softer?
- Is the baby obviously satisfied?
- Does the baby settle well after the feed?
- Can you hear/see the baby swallow?

7.5.2 How to make a nursing supplementer

A simple nursing supplementer can be made very easily (see Fig. 7.8). Use a cup or bottle of milk, with the end of a size 0.4 or 0.6 feeding tube placed in the milk, and the tip of the tube secured just above the mother's areola, with the tip very slightly over the end of the nipple (as previously described). The milk is then obtained when the baby begins to feed from the breast.

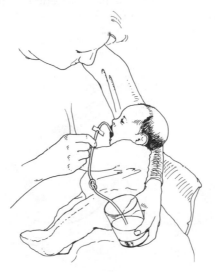

Fig. 7.8 A 'home-made' nursing supplementer.

7.5.3   Long-term use of the nursing supplementer

A mother who is not able to produce sufficient of her own milk for her baby can still breastfeed using a nursing supplementer. She may find having at least three supplementers will be useful. She can wear one of them under her clothes, so that she is always ready for when her baby wishes to breastfeed. The milk will be at the right temperature when the baby suckles. The remaining two supplementers can be kept in the refrigerator until required. The formula milk used can be made up in the mornings so that the mother always has milk available.

7.6   Syringes and droppers

These are not often used to administer extra fluids, although they are occasionally used to give drugs. It is important, if they are used, that the syringe or dropper is squeezed as the baby is sucking, but not swallowing. The milk or other fluid should be aimed towards the inside of the baby's cheek rather than towards the tongue or back of his throat. To prevent aspiration, which is always a danger when a baby is unable to pace his own intake, the baby should be held or sitting in an upright semi-reclining position, not flat.

A syringe may also be used to encourage breastfeeding in the following way (see Fig. 7.9):

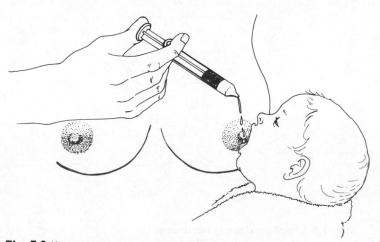

Fig. 7.9 *Using a syringe to encourage breastfeeding.*

1. A quantity of expressed breastmilk is put into a 10 or 20 ml syringe.
2. The baby is positioned at the breast, with his mouth close to the mother's nipple and areola.
3. A little breastmilk is squeezed on to the nipple area from the syringe.
4. The baby is encouraged to lick the milk from the nipple.
5. If he begins to open his mouth widely, his mother may attach him to the breast if possible. The milk from the syringe should be stopped at this point or just trickled on to the breast very slowly. If successful attachment is achieved then using the syringe can be discontinued.

This method may be useful for: babies who refuse or are reluctant to attach to the breast; preterm babies who do not have the strength to suckle effectively, but are able to lick and swallow the milk trickled on to the breast; mothers whose let-down reflex is temporarily inhibited for whatever reason.

7.7 Finger 'assessment' of feeding

This is a simple and effective diagnostic method of assessing a baby's ability to suck and swallow efficiently. It allows assessment of tongue movement, and the baby's ability to cope with milk boluses. However, it should **only** be used for this purpose where conventional feeding methods continually fail.

Note the movement of the tongue. It should move in a rhythmical way from the front to the back and form a furrow around the finger (or breast/nipple). An uncoordinated tongue may be haphazard in its movement, creating pressure on parts of the palate that are inappropriate for sucking or for eliciting the swallow reflex. Where this happens, cup-feeding may help to correct the problem. Gentle agitation with the tip of the finger on the junction of the hard and soft palate should cause a swallow response. Milk **should not** be given unless a swallow reflex is present.

'Finger assessment' may be useful when a baby is admitted for 'poor feeding' and does not appear to improve with any conventional method of feeding.

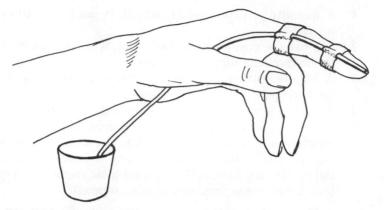

Fig. 7.10 *The position of a feeding tube for 'finger assessment of feeding'.*

7.7.1   Method

1. Wash hands carefully.
2. Fill a cup with the amount of milk the baby is due to have.
3. Place one end of a size 4 or 6 gastric tube on the pad of the index finger, the other in the cup of milk.
4. Fix the tube at the first joint of the finger with tape (see Fig. 7.10).
5. At the same time as putting your finger in the baby's mouth, with the pad directed towards the hard palate, hold the cup slightly higher than the baby so that, as soon as he begins to suck, the milk will flow. Once the milk is in the tube, put the cup in a convenient place.

'Finger feeding' is a feeding technique used in some parts of the world. It is primarily used to help babies who do not attach to the breast after birth,[12] for breast refusal and as a temporary feeding method for mothers with sore nipples.[13] However, the sucking technique used by the baby is very similar to the technique of bottle-feeding. It should, therefore, be used with extreme caution if breastfeeding is the desired outcome.

7.8   The bottle

It is better to **avoid using bottles altogether**, if a baby is to be breastfed. When a situation arises in hospital where an alternative oral method of feeding, or supplementation **is** required, health professionals can use a cup,[14] or a spoon, and a mother may additionally use a nursing supplementer or a syringe.

However, if it is **the wish** of a mother to go home breast- and bottle-feeding, it is important to find out why exclusive breastfeeding is not possible. For example, perhaps the mother is going back to work, and believes she must get her baby used to a bottle; perhaps she feels family pressure to 'share' the baby's feeding or perhaps she feels apprehensive at the idea of the baby being entirely dependent on her. Whatever the reason, make sure the mother is aware that alternatives to the bottle **do exist** and can be used safely. If she is returning to work, it is worth talking through the options: such as finding a child minder near her work place so that she can breastfeed during the day or considering creche facilities. If more mothers ask for these facilities, the more likely they are to be made available!

If a mother is certain that she wishes to introduce bottles, find out if expressed breastmilk or formula milk are to be used. If she wishes to use expressed breastmilk she needs to be confident in her skill of expressing and know how to hand express. Even if she does not intend to use this method; it can be useful if her hand or electric pump fails. She also needs to know how to store the milk safely. If the mother is going to use formula milk, she should be aware that her own milk supply may diminish, if she does not express regularly and gets less breast stimulation.

Some babies will also develop a preference for either the breast or the bottle, therefore, it is important that a baby is **established** at the breast **before** bottle (or a dummy) is introduced.

If a mother is having problems with breastfeeding, which do not appear to respond to help, she should be encouraged to continue breastfeeding whenever possible, even if a bottle is introduced. She should not feel under pressure to feed only by bottle or only by breast, particularly if this results in breastfeeding being abandoned unnecessarily. It is possible for some babies to feed by both methods – and it is better to have some breastfeeds than none at all. Explain the situation to the mother's health visitor and/or community midwife. Also encourage the mother to contact her local National Childbirth Trust, La Leche League or Association of Breastfeeding Mothers breastfeeding counsellor to ensure she has consistent support and advice after discharge.

7.8.1   Preterm babies and bottle-feeding

Preterm babies who are to be breastfed should **not** be given bottles. It is important they learn to breastfeed without being confused by using another sucking pattern.

7.8.2   Bottle teats, dummies and the vulnerable baby

Permission (preferably written) **should be obtained** from the parents before a bottle or dummy is given to **any** baby who is to be breastfed.

If a baby is to be bottle-fed, he can be given a dummy quite safely, without the danger of teaching an inappropriate feeding technique. Both dummies and nipple shields encourage the same pattern of sucking movements as bottle teats, because they are static in the mouth, unlike the breast which is softer and more pliable.

If a breastfed baby is admitted to the unit with 'feeding problems', a dummy may simply encourage an inappropriate sucking action or reinforce incorrect tongue movements, thus making the problem worse.

For mothers of babies with difficulties in feeding directly from the breast, i.e. cleft lip and/or palate, expressed breastmilk can be given by bottle, if breastfeeding is not considered possible, using special teats, which allow the milk flow to be regulated.

7.9   Mixed breast- and bottle-feeding

Some babies **are** able to feed from both the breast and bottle without any apparent difficulty. When establishment at the breast has taken place before introduction to a bottle or dummy has occurred, a baby appears less likely to have as many problems with the two different sucking techniques. However, it is impossible to know which babies will manage the two methods of feeding without any problems and which babies will go on to refuse to breastfeed, or bottle-feed. A period of time, for example, at least 1 month, should be allowed to elapse before introducing a bottle to a clinically well baby, born at term. The period of time suggested is arbitrary but is long enough to allow a baby to become well established at the breast first. It is ideal to delay introducing a bottle to a preterm baby until he has reached at least 37 weeks post-conception age or is well established at the breast, which may be later or earlier than 37 weeks. Preterm babies appear to be more susceptible than term babies to problems of adapting to different techniques of sucking.[15]

Gestational age at birth and level of maturity at the time of the introduction of oral feeding may substantially influence whether a baby can feed successfully by both breast and bottle. Some **term** babies appear to develop a **'preference'** for a bottle teat. They are capable of doing either and can distinguish the different feeding techniques for suckling at the breast or sucking on a bottle teat. They may eventually prefer one to the other. Some **preterm** babies appear to become genuinely **'confused'** about how to feed from the breast or from a bottle teat, especially if they are introduced to different feeding techniques before breastfeeding has been established.

Similarly, a baby who is ill at birth or shortly afterwards, regardless of gestational age and who is able to feed orally, may use only one method of feeding and refuse the other method. If, for example, bottle feeding has been the dominant method of feeding, then the baby may reject breastfeeding and vice versa. A term baby who is ill at birth or becomes ill in the early postnatal period may temporarily lose the mature co-ordination of the 'suck', 'swallow' and 'breathing' reflexes necessary for effective nutritive feeding. This baby may relapse into feeding in the way he finds the most familiar.

There is no evidence to show that different-shaped teats make it easier for a baby to adapt to breastfeeding. Where mothers want to have the opportunity to feed with both methods, different teats, which make the baby open his mouth wider or remove the milk by using compression should be examined. These teats may also have some advantages for the exclusively bottle-fed baby.

References

1 Roy RN, Pollnitz RP, Hamilton JR and Chance GW (1977) Impaired assimilation of nasojejunal feeds in healthy low-birth-weight newborn infants. *J Pediatr* **90**: 431–434.

2 Martenez FE, Desai ID, Davidson AGF, Nakai S and Radcliffe A (1987) Ultrasound homogenization of expressed human milk to prevent fat loss during tube feeding. *J Pediatr Gastroenterol Nutrition* **6**: 593–597.

3   Kelnar JH and Harvey D (1987) Delay of development of suck reflex in infants. In *The Sick Newborn Baby*, 2nd edn. Kelnar JH and Harvey D (eds). London: Balliere Tindall, pp. 134–159.
4   Selley WG and Boxall J (1986) A new way to treat sucking and swallowing difficulties in babies. *Lancet*, i: 1182–1184.
5   Hamosh M, Bitman J, Fink CS, Freed LM, York CM, Wood DL, Mehta NR and Hamosh P (1985) Lipid composition of preterm human milk and its digestion by the infant. In *Composition and Physiological Properties of Human Milk*. Schaub J (ed.). Oxford: Elsevier Science Publishers, pp. 153–162.
6   Coulter McBride M and Coulter Danner S (1987) Sucking disorders in neurologically impaired infants: assessment and facilitation of breastfeeding. In *Clin Perinatol* March: *Breastfeeding*, Lawrence R (ed.), pp. 109–130.
7   Giroux JD, Sizun J and Alix D (1991) L'alimentation a la tasse chez le nouveau-ne. *Arch Fr Pediatr* **48**: 737–740.
8   Lang S, Lawrence CJ and L'E Orme R (1994) Cup feeding: an alternative method of infant feeding. *Arch Child Dis* **71**: 365–369.
9   Lang S (1994) Cup-feeding: an alternative method. *Midwives Chronicle* **107**: 171–176.
10   Smith LJ (1986) Neonatal fat digestion and lingual lipase. *Acta Paediatr Scand* **75**: 913–918.
11   Lebenthal E, Heitlinger L and Milla PJ (1988) Prenatal and perinatal development of the gastrointestinal tract. In *Harries Paediatric Gastroenterology*, 2nd edn. Milla PJ, Muller DPR (eds). Edinburgh: Churchill Livingstone, pp. 3–29.
12   Auerbach KG, Riordan J and Countryman BA (1993) The breastfeeding process. In *Breastfeeding and Human Lactation*. Riordan J and Auerbach KG (eds). London: Jones & Bartlett, pp. 221–222.
13   Newman J (1990) Breastfeeding problems associated with the early introduction of bottles and pacifiers. *J Human Lact* **6**: 59–63.
11   Armstrong H (1986) Are feeding bottles ever needed? *1986: Breastfeeding Briefs*. Prepared by the Geneva Infant Feeding Association, member of the International Baby Food Action Network (IBFAN), September 1986.
15   Lang S (1995) *Feeding and Growth Patterns of Infants in a Neonatal Unit*. Unpublished M.Phil. Thesis, University of Exeter.

8 Breastfeeding and common drugs

8.1 Breastfeeding and drugs

Always ask a mother who is breastfeeding or who intends to breastfeed if she is taking any medicines. There is an extensive list in the British National Formulary (BNF) on drugs and breastfeeding (a copy of this is available in all hospital clinical areas), and in the World Health Organization's (WHO) *Annex on Breastfeeding and Maternal Medication Recommendations for Drugs in the Essential Drugs List.*[1]* Either of these documents should be consulted whenever there is any doubt over a drug given to a lactating mother.

Breastmilk is generally free from contamination, although certain drugs and other substances can be passed into the milk via the mother's bloodstream. It is important, therefore, to make sure **any** 'medicines' or 'remedies', from any source, are compatable with breastfeeding. Treatments based on homeopathy, aromatherapy or other less obvious practices should also be asked about, particularly because several 'remedies' are now bought 'over the counter' without any consultation with a 'specialist'. It is quite possible, if a mother is experiencing a problem with her milk supply or the baby is refusing her breast, that she may be taking some form of 'medicine' without realizing it could have a negative effect on her lactation in some way – even if it only makes the taste of the milk less palatable to her baby!

Remember that:

---

* *This can be obtained with the training materials for the WHO (Breastfeeding Counselling: A Training Course) from World Health Organization, Secretariat, Division of Diarrhoeal and Acute Respiratory Disease Control, World Health Organization, CH-1211 Geneva 27, Switzerland.*

- Mothers should have no drugs during the nursing period unless prescribed by a doctor.
- The mother must remember to inform her doctor that she is breastfeeding if she needs any form of medication during this period. A prepared form, on which her doctor can write down any drugs the mother is prescribed, and which can be kept with her baby's notes would be useful, particularly if the medication is not well known.
- Ask the mother if she is on any drugs and their name/s. Check for yourself if it is safe for her to take them while breastfeeding. Check with a doctor on the unit or with the pharmacy, if you are unsure or worried.

8.1.1 Some common drugs to avoid

The combined contraceptive pill

The combined contraceptive pill, containing oestrogen and progesterone, should be avoided during lactation. Products containing oestrogen are known to cause significant reductions in milk volume – one study found this to be by as much as 40%.[2,3] Therefore, if low milk supply suddenly becomes a problem at around 6 weeks, check whether a mother has begun taking the combined pill. It is important, if she **has resumed** taking oral contraception, to ensure she is taking the **'mini-pill'** (containing progesterone only). However, this is not without its drawbacks either, for evidence suggests that progesterone can cause a reduction in the fat content of breastmilk.[3]

Caffeine

Although tea, coffee and Coca-Cola are not drugs in the accepted sense – caffeine is! Caffeine can pass into breastmilk, but this does not usually cause problems. However, if a mother is accustomed to drinking several cups of strong coffee (6–8) per day, it may cause restlessness in her baby. If a mother cannot give up any drinks containing caffeine, advise her to have her drink shortly after breastfeeding and, if possible, to drink weaker coffee or tea. Using a decaffeinated brand of coffee or tea will lessen, but not totally eliminate, her caffeine consumption.

Nicotine

Smoking should be discontinued if at all possible.[4,5] Nicotine is potentially hazardous to a baby in much the same way as it is to children and adults. Where a mother is unable to give up cigarettes, she should smoke **after breastfeeding**, not before. Smoking can, through vasoconstriction, cause considerable diminishing of the milk supply. Encourage mothers to smoke less. Passive intake of smoke is also hazardous and should be avoided whenever possible.

8.2   Breastfeeding and maternal medication

The following information gives a brief outline, based on the advice of the WHO,[1] on drugs prescribed to a mother and breastfeeding.

8.2.1   Medication with contraindications to breastfeeding

1. Anti-cancer drugs.
2. Radioactive substances (in this case breastfeeding may be stopped for a temporary period only).

8.2.2   Medication with which breastfeeding can be continued

1. In the following case, side effects are possible and the baby should be monitored for drowsiness:

    •   Psychiatric drugs and anticonvulsants.

2. An alternative to the following drugs should be used if possible:

    •   Chloramphenicol.
    •   Tetracyclines.
    •   Metronidazole.
    •   Quinolone antibiotics (e.g. ciprofloacin).

3. These drugs may decrease the milk supply, therefore alternatives should be used whenever possible:

- Oestrogen.
- Thiazide diuretics.
- Ergometrine.

4. The baby should be monitored for jaundice if the following drugs are taken by the mother:

- Sulphonamides.
- Co-trimaxazole.
- Fansidar.
- Dapsone.

5. These drugs are safe in normally prescribed dosages; however, the baby should be monitored when they are taken by the mother.

- Analgesics: short courses of paracetamol, acetylsalicylic acid, ibuprofen and occasional doses of morphine and pethidine.
- Antibiotics: penicillin, ampicillan, cloxacillan, erythromycin.
- Anti-histamines.
- Antacids.
- Digoxin.
- Insulin.
- Bronchodilators (e.g. Salbutamol).
- Corticosteroids.
- Anti-helminthes.
- Chloroquine.
- Anti-tuberculars.

6. Nutritional supplements of iron, iodine and vitamins can also be taken in the prescribed dosages.

N.B. Whenever possible, drugs should be **avoided** during the breastfeeding period.

References

1 WHO (1993) *Annex on Breastfeeding and Maternal Medication Recommendations for Drugs in the Essential Drugs List.* Geneva: World Health Organization.
2 Tankeyoon M, Dusitsin N, Chalapati S *et al.* (1984) Effects of hor-

monal contraception on milk volume and infant growth. *Contraception* **30**: 505–522.

3 WHO (1989) Infant feeding: the physiological basis. Akre J (ed.) *Bulletin* **67** (Suppl.): 41–54.

4 Carlson DE (1988) Maternal diseases associated with intra-uterine growth retardation. *Perinatol* **12**: 17–22.

5 Fox H (1991) A contemporary view of the human placenta. *Midwifery* **17**: 31–39.

9 Recommendations for the support of breastfeeding

9.1 Recommendations for the support of breastfeeding on a neonatal or specialist paediatric unit

Lactation management should have an important place in the overall plan of care within a neonatal or similar specialist unit.

9.1.1 Staff education

In order to help the mothers and their babies in our neonatal and other specialist units to succeed in breastfeeding, the staff who care for them have to be both skilled and knowledgeable. The following suggestions aim to make the process of education available to all members of staff, and encourage units to have a practical approach to lactation management and training.

1. A comprehensive and practical set of breastfeeding guidelines, appropriate to the needs of babies on a neonatal or paediatric unit or in any other specialist area, should be available to all staff, nursing and medical. These guidelines should incorporate or reflect the breastfeeding policy or guidelines of the maternity unit, so that the mothers are given consistent advice by the staff of all clinical areas. (Because of the different backgrounds of the staff who work in various specialist units, it is important that the guidelines do not assume knowledge of lactation which may not be present.)
2. A set of up-to-date reference materials (books, slides and videos) on lactation and infant feeding should be available

to staff, for private study, reference and to guide the policies of a particular clinical area.

3. Regular in-service training sessions should be held which update staff and ensure practical skills are continually assessed (in the same way as other skills relating to neonatal nursing are assessed). These could be organized between the maternity, paediatric and neonatal units to encourage co-operation between the units, and to provide a forum for sharing the different experiences of breastfeeding of their staff members.

4. Basic lactational management and skill training should be given in all the training and orientation programmes for new staff choosing to work in neonatal, maternity or paediatric units.

5. To ensure all neonatal and paediatric unit staff receive adequate practical training in lactation, a work book could be used in which a number of practical skills are recorded. For example, **all** staff to observe at least 15 normal complete breastfeeds on a **maternity** unit; observe 5 mothers hand expressing and 5 mothers using a mechanical pump; observe 15 mothers and their preterm babies in the process of establishing breastfeeding; any abnormal breast physiology observed could be recorded. A second section could be devoted to assisting mothers and their babies. This booklet could be part of the basic training requirements alongside any other similar course requirements in the speciality. (Midwives, for example, already use such a book throughout their basic training to record number of antenatal examinations performed, deliveries observed and conducted, postnatal checks undertaken.)

6. Unit audits of the effectiveness of feeding policies should be undertaken at regular intervals. These may be conducted alongside other audits, which are already undertaken, and any changes to policies made if necessary. Records of mothers' feeding intentions and outcomes should be held.

7. Neonatal and paediatric unit staff should be aware of the 'Baby Friendly Hospital Initiative' (BFHI)* and display the 'Ten Steps to Successful Breastfeeding' in the unit. They should encourage the maternity unit to aim towards BFHI status. The self-appraisal tool, which is available with the

---

* Information about the Baby Friendly Hospital Initiative can be obtained from: UNICEF, 20 Guilford Street, London WC1N 1DZ. The self-appraisal tool can also be obtained from UNICEF, at this address.

information pack on the BFHI, could be used to raise awareness among the staff of the areas of practice that require strengthening.

9.1.2 The neonatal unit

In addition to increasing staff awareness of the important theoretical and practical aspects of lactation, the neonatal or paediatric units have to promote a positive atmosphere towards breastfeeding. This can be achieved in the following ways:

1. On each working shift, one member of staff could be designated to be responsible for the care of lactating and breastfeeding mothers.
2. By adopting a 'no-bottle' policy for babies to be breastfed, unless bottles are specifically requested by the parents.
3. By having a room available for mothers who wish to express or breastfeed in private, preferably with facilities for making drinks, or the provision of adequate screens for mothers who wish to express or breastfeed in private, when a specific room is not available.
4. By making general information about breastfeeding and other feeding methods available to parents. This information could be put on a noticeboard for parents to read at their leisure. Pamphlets from the various support groups should be readily available, such as those from the National Childbirth Trust (NCT), the La Leche League and the Association of Breastfeeding Mothers, and also specialist leaflets, for example, from CLAPA (the Cleft Lip and Palate Association). Posters are available from the Royal College of Midwives and the UNICEF BFHI for the UK. Alternatively, photographs taken on the particular unit could form the basis of the information given. Responsibility for the board could be rotated among the staff.
5. The Kardex or nursing notes relating to the baby's care should contain a section documenting the advice and practical help in lactation given to a mother. This could form part of any care plan, so that it is updated on a daily basis.
6. An infant feeding specialist is recommended for the neonatal unit. Their role could incorporate the breastfeeding needs of the maternity and paediatric units. They could be a resource person for both staff and parents, and provide

support and help to the community midwives, health visitors, practice nurses and general practitioners.

7. By the full implemention of the WHO International Code of Marketing of Breastmilk Substitutes.[1] Branded milks should not be on display, and no posters from formula milk companies should be used to promote either breast or bottle feeding. No cot cards, growth charts, note pads, diary covers, pens or other material should be used supporting formula milk company logos.

8. The provision of alternative feeding devices, e.g. the nursing supplementer and cups.

It may seem idealistic to suggest that more staff should be employed, i.e. a feeding specialist, to help mothers achieve success in breastfeeding. However, breastfeeding has to be seen in the context of long-term benefits rather than short-term gains. If, for example, fewer mothers suffer breast cancer or hip fractures, and fewer babies are admitted to paediatric units with gastrointestinal illness or *otitis media*, then it is an investment in the future health of the population of a Trust area.

9.1.3 Helping the parents

Further measures, which would specifically help parents and particularly mothers, include:

1. The provision of information booklets based on the unit breastfeeding guidelines, which give clear and simple information. This information should be available in different languages if appropriate. (Similar booklets could be available on bottle-feeding for parents wishing to bottle-feed for they also need to be taught to use bottles correctly.)

2. A designated member of staff (not necessarily the person looking after the baby) should give the mother the help and advice she requires on lacation, as soon as possible after delivery. To ensure continuity, this member of staff should, where possible, provide the advice to the mother throughout her baby's stay on the unit.

3. A support group for breastfeeding mothers (and their partners) would help overcome some of the feelings of isolation these mothers can experience. This could be organized initially by the staff of a unit or one of the volun-

tary breastfeeding counsellor organizations. It could gradually be given over to the parents themselves to run. It is helpful for this to take place in the hospital and for a member of staff also to attend – to offer any help or advice, which may be sought.

4. Mothers who are expressing breastmilk or breastfeeding require the support of a range of people. Breastfeeding counsellors from the NCT or La Leche League can provide continuing support, both while the baby is in hospital and after discharge. Therefore, the mother should be put in touch with such a counsellor during the baby's period in hospital.

5. Parents could be asked to give written permission for the use of dummies/pacifiers or bottles to be used if the baby is to be breastfed.

References

1   IBFAN(1993) *Protecting Infant Health: A Health Worker's Guide to the International Code of Marketing of Breastmilk Substitutes*, 7th edn. Penang, Malaysia: IBFAN.

Appendix: Breastfeeding support

Breastfeeding support groups

National Childbirth Trust, Breastfeeding Promotion Group, Alexandra House, Oldham Terrace, Acton, London W3 6NH. Tel. (0181) 992 8637.
La Leche League, Breastfeeding Help and Information, BM 3424, London WC1 6XX. Tel. (0171) 242 1278.
Association of Breastfeeding Mothers, 26 Holmshaw Close, London SE26 4TH. Tel. (0181) 778 4769.

Other useful addresses

Twins and Multiple Births Association, 41 Fortuna Way, Grimsby, South Humberside, DN37 9SJ.
Cleft Lip and Palate Association, Hospital for Sick Children, Great Ormond Street, London WC1N 3JH. Tel. (0171) 405 9200.
UNICEF Baby Friendly Initiative, 20 Guilford Street, London WC1N 1DZ. Tel. (0171) 405 8400 ext 430.
Baby Milk Action Coalition, 5 St Andrews Place, Cambridge CB2 3AX. Tel. (01223) 464420.
British Homeopathic Association, 27a Devonshire Street, London W1N 2RJ.
British Council of Complementary Therapies, PO Box 194, London SE16 1Q2. Tel. (0171) 237 5165.

Useful literature

Books

Akre, J (ed.) (1989) *Infant Feeding – The Physiological Basis*, WHO Bulletin, vol. 67, (Suppl.). ISBN 92–4–068670–3

Helsing E and Savage-King F (1985) *Breastfeeding in Practice*. Oxford: Oxford University Press. ISBN: 0–19–261485–1

Henschel D and Inch S (1996) *Breastfeeding: A Guide for Midwives*. Hale, Cheshire: Books for Midwives Press. ISBN: 1–898507–12–0

La Leche League (1981) *The Womanly Art of Breast Feeding*. Franklin, IL: La Leche League International.

La Leche League International (1992) *The Breastfeeding Answer Book*. Franklin Park, IL: La Leche League. ISBN: 0–912500–33–6

Lawrence R (1994) *Breastfeeding: A Guide for the Medical Profession*, 4th edn. London: Mosby. ISBN: 0–8016–6858–1

Minchin M (1989) *Breastfeeding Matters*. Almadale: Allen & Unwin. ISBN: 0–86861–810–1

Palmer G (1988) *The Politics of Breastfeeding*. London: Pandora Press. ISBN: 0–86358–220–6

Renfrew M, Fisher C and Armes S (1990) *Best Feeding*. Celestial Arts. ISBN: 0–889087–571–5

Riordan J (1991) *A Practical Guide to Breastfeeding*. London: Jones & Bartlett. ISBN: 0–86720–448–6

Riordan J and Auerbach K (1993) *Breastfeeding and Human Lactation*. London: Jones & Bartlett. ISBN: 0–86720–343–9

Royal College of Midwives (1991) *Successful Breastfeeding*, 2nd edn. Edinburgh: Churchill Livingstone. ISBN: 1–870822–01–3

Stanway P and Stanway A (1988) *Breast is Best*. London: Pan Books. ISBN: 0330–28110–0

WHO Working Group on Infant Growth (1994) *An Evaluation of Infant Growth*. Geneva: Nutrition Unit, WHO

Other literature

Breastfeeding Abstracts: Published quarterly by La Leche League International. Obtained from the national organization for a small annual subscription.

Breastfeeding Briefs: Published quarterly by GIFA, Box 157, 1211 Geneva 19, Switzerland at UNICEF national offices.

Index

Note: Page references in *italics* refer to figures; those in **bold** refer to main discussion

abscess, breast 83, 85–6, 105
  signs 85
  treatment 86
acupuncture 95
adoption
  relactation for 105
  relactation and use of nursing
    supplementer 151
after pains 4
allergic conditions 3
alternative and supplementary
    feeding methods, types of
    126
amylase 11
analgesia, maternal, effect on
    feeding 16
antibiotics
  complementary feeds and 70
  effect on baby of maternal 85
  feeding babies having 38
  intake of colostrum by baby
    receiving 54
  for mastitis 85
arachidonic acid (AA) 10
areola *see* nipples
Association of Breastfeeding
    Mothers 157, 168
attachment, breast **30–2**, *31*
  difficulty in 33–4
  results of poor 32, *32*
Ayurvedic medicine 9

Baby Friendly Hospital Initiative
    167–8
back massage **60–3**, *61*, *62*
Bell's palsy 118–19

benefits of breastfeeding
  to baby 3
  to mother 1, 3–4
bile salt-stimulated lipase (BSSL)
    10, 141
bilirubin 9
  see also jaundice
blocked ducts and lobes **82–4**
  prevention 84
  signs of 82–3
  treatment 83–4
bottle-feeding 156–8
  bottle teats and dummies 158
  breastfeeding after 34
  in cleft lip/palate 116
  mixed breast- and 158–9
  preterm babies and 158
bowels 132–3
  colour and consistency of
    stools 132
  frequency of action 133
  warning signs 132–3
breast cancer, premenopause 3
breast, lactating, anatomy and
    physiology 4–7, *5*
breast lumps 105
breast massage 62, **65–9**, 94
  to encourage milk supply 56,
    60, 122
  reason for 65–6
  technique 66–9, *67*
  two-handed 67–8, *68*
  using fingertips 68–9, *69*
breast pads 98
breast reduction 104
breast shell 71–2, *72*

breast support 77, *78*
breast surgery 104–5
  inadequate milk production
    and 93
  use of nursing supplementer
    151
breastmilk
  benefits of 4
  colour 7
  composition of 2, 7–13, 57
  contamination 57
  effect of storage container on
    52–3, 57
  frequency of feeds 37–8
  mature 7
  term and preterm 9–13
  transitional 7
  see also breastmilk production;
    colostrum
breastmilk production **92–8**
  appearance of stages 7
  excess 96–8
  inadequate 92–6
  leaking breasts 97–8, *97*, *98*
  physical factors causing low
    93
  remedies 93–6
  sequence *8*
  sufficient 38–9
breastpumps
  double pumping 55, *56*, 65
  hand 6
  frequency of use 53, 94
  length of expression 53
  mechanical 6, **52–6**
  technique 54–6
  types 65
  volume of milk produced by
    53–4
  weaning off from using 63–5,
    97
  when to use 52–4
breathing reflex 15, 16

cabbage leaves, use in soothing
    breasts 75, 84, 85
Caesarean section
  expressing milk following 52
  feeding position following 29
caffeine 108, 162
calcium in breastmilk 12

Calendula cream 79
Candida albicans 76, 133
Cannon teat 116
carbohydrate in breastmilk 11
cardiac problems
  breastfeeding baby with
    119–20
  effect on feeding 16
  length of feed 35
casein 11
Cleft Lip and Palate Association
    (CLAPA) 116, 168
cleft lip/palate 15, **111–18**
  cleft lip 111–12
  cleft lip and palate 111–12, 114
  cleft palate 112–14, *113*
  cup-feeding in 143, 147
  establishment of breastfeeding
    114–16
  feeding position 25, 27–8, 29
  general advice 117–18
  hand expression and 43
  if breastfeeding is not
    established 116
  support groups 116–17
  use of nipple shield 88
clothing, securing 23, *24*
colic 128
colostrum 8–9, 44
  defrosting 53
  expression of 50, 53
  laxative effect of 132
  reduction of development of
    jaundice by 125
  volume produced 58
  weight loss caused by 103
containers, storage 56–7
continuous positive airways
    pressure (CPAP) 142
continuous pump feeds 137–8
contraceptive pill 95
  combined 162
  deficiency of vitamin B6 with
    long-term use 12
cup-feeding 15, 141, **143–50**
  advantages 143
  cleft lip/palate and 147
  cup types 149
  disadvantages 143
  general reasons for using
    143–4
  holding position 149, *150*

of jaundiced baby 126
method 149–50
as oral stimulation 40–1
of pre-term baby 123–4, *143*, 145–6
quantities taken 148–9
of term baby 146–7
type of milk 150
when and how to use 144–7

Daktarin 133
Dancer position 33, *33*
defrosting milk 57–8
demand feeding 38, 74, 93
dental caries 3
dental plate 137, 139
diet, maternal 107–8
disabled mother, feeding position 29
docosahexaenoic acid (DHA) 10
domperidone 95
double pumping 55, *56*, 65
Down's syndrome 15, 43
use of nursing supplementer 151
drip catchers 71–2
droppers 154–5
drugs **161–4**
to avoid 162–3
contraindications 163
decreasing milk supply 163–4
effect on breastmilk 52
maternal medication 163–4
side effects 163
dummies 40
breastfeeding after using 34
inappropriate use 148
as oral stimulation 41–2

emotional upset, effect of, on milk supply 54
engorgement 65, 74–6
initial fullness 74–5
as result of poor attachment 32
epidermal growth factor (EGF) 8
Escherichia coli 9
expression of breastmilk
back massage 60–3, *61*, *62*
direct 36, 43, 117, 141–3, *142*
of fat-rich hind-milk 99–102

formula 100–2
prevention of engorgement 75
prolonged 58–65
promotion of weight gain and growth in preterm babies 100
promotion of weight gain in breastfeeding babies 102
reducing long-term problems 59–60
sequence of use 58
see also breastpumps; hand expression
eye infection 84

fat
adhesion to storage containers 57
content of breastmilk 9–11
fatty acids 10
feed
frequency 37–8
length of 34–6
night 37
prolonged 35–6
remedies for prolonged 35–6
feeding ability
development of 13–15
factors affecting efficiency of 15–17
fertility, return of 3
finger 'assessment' of feeding 136, 155–6, *156*
finger feeding 156
flexi-shield 55, *55*
fluids, maternal intake of 107–8
folic acid 12
food poisoning 9
fore-milk
fat content 10
hand expression of 44
frenulum as cause of tongue tie 111
frozen milk 57–8
fructose 11

gag reflex 14
galactase 17
galactosaemia 17
galactose 11

gastric tube 14
  1–2 hourly bolus 138–9, 140–1
  3 hourly 141
  breastfeeding and 139–41
  continuous 137–8, 140
  in preterm baby with 124, 126
  sucking and 39–40
  using formula milk 141
  in ventilated baby 124
  see also nasal gastric tube; oral
    gastric tube
geranium leaves 79
growth
  normal 102
  periods of rapid 37–8, 92

Habermann teat 116, 119
haemorrhagic disease of the
    newborn 12
hand expression 6, 36, **43–52**
  of both breasts 48, *49*
  position of fingers 46, *46*
  practical instruction 51–2, *51*
  preparation 45–6
  principles 46–7
  reasons for teaching 43–4
  single session of 49–50
  teaching 50–2
  technique 45–50
  timing and frequency 44–5
  two-hand technique 48, *48*
  variations 48
hind-milk, fat content 10
hip fractures 3
HIV 133–4
Hodgkin's disease 3
hypoglycaemia **129–32**
  at-risk babies 129–30
  definition 129–30
  high-risk baby 131–2
  high-risk factors 130
  low-risk baby 130–1
  low-risk factors 130
  symptoms 130

immunoglobulins 8, 11
  IgA, secretory 8
  IgG 8
  IgM 8
iron in breastmilk 13

jaundice 9, 125–7
  breastmilk 127
  frequency of feeds 37
  maternal drugs and 164
  pathological or haemolytic 126
  phototherapy 126–7
  physiological or idiopathic 125
  prolonged feeding 36
  reducing development of 125
  supplementary feeding 71
juvenile onset diabetes 3

La Leche League 116, 157, 168,
    170
lactase 11
lactase deficiency 17
lactation
  artificial stimulation of 6–7
  inhibition of 6–7
  initiation of 5–6
  see also breastmilk production;
    lactation management
lactation management
  helping the parents 169–70
  neonatal unit 168–9
  staff education 166–8
lactiferous sinuses 4, 47
Lactobacillus bifidus 11
'Lactofelicine' 9
lactose 11
lamb's teat 116
let-down reflex 6, 60
  effect of tension on 92
lipases 9, 10, 14, 40, 124, 144
lipoprotein lipase (LPL) 10
Listeria 9
lymphoma 3

magnesium 12
malocclusion of teeth 3
mastectomy, bilateral 104
mastitis 65, 75, 83, 84–5
  position for feeding 25
  preventing 44
  signs 84–5
  treatment 85
meconium 132
metoclopramide 95, 106
milk *see* breastmilk
milk, maternal intake of 108
mini-pill 95, 162

monolauryl 9
Mother tincture (*Urtica urens*)
 95
multiple births *see* twins;
 triplets

nasal gastric tube 137
 avoiding 139
 during phototherapy 126
 occuring *140*
National Childbirth Trust 116,
 157, 168, 170
necrotizing enterocolitis 3, 137
nicotine 163
night feeds 69
nipple
 cracked 32, 76, 78–9
 effect of shape on feeding
  efficiency 16
 massage of 60, 66, 95
 pink/red with no cracks 76–7
 removal from 76, 77
 soothing with milk 44, 77
 sore 32, 76–9
 see also nipples, inverted or
  flat
nipple shield 77, **86–90**, *87*
 avoiding use of 86–8
 to reduce milk supply 97
 use of 88–9
 weaning baby off 89–90
nipples, inverted or flat 16,
 79–82, *79*
 attachment of baby 80, *81*
 low milk production and 93
 management 80–2
 syringe method of treatment
  81, *81*
 use of breast shells 72
nursing chairs 22, *23*
nursing supplementer 87, 90,
 150–4, *151*
 following breast surgery 105
 home-made 153, *153*
 in jaundiced baby 127
 long-term use 154
 method 152–3
 situations for using 150–2
 use in increasing milk supply
  94
Nystatin 133

obdurator 129
oligosaccharides 11
oral gastric tube 129, 131
 in phototherapy 118
 securing *132*
oral stimulation 38–42
otitis media 3
 in baby with cleft lip/palate
  111
ovarian cancer 3
oxygen therapy, baby dependent
 on 22, 119–20, *120*
oxytocin 3, 6, 24, 60, 95, 106
oxytocin nasal spray 95

pethidine, effect on feeding 16
phosphorus 12
phototherapy 70, 126–7
Pierre Robin syndrome 15, 31
positioning **25–30**
 in feeding twins 30
 laying down 29
 monitoring and oxygen
  therapy 21–2
 in overproduction of milk 96,
  97
 preparation for 22–5
 in tandem feeding 30
 traditional 28–9, *29*
 underarm 26–8, *26*
premature rupture of
  membranes (PROM) 54
preterm babies
 feeding position 122
 frequency of feeds 38
 length of feeds 35
 milk supply 121
 overcoming problems 122–4
 sucking pattern 122–3
progesterone 5–6
prolactin 3, 4, 6, 24, 37, 95, 105
protein, milk 11
psychological benefits of
  breastfeeding 4
pyloric stenosis 15

relactation **105–7**
 if breastmilk has been
  produced previously 106
 if breastmilk has never been
  produced 107

relactation (*cont.*)
  use of nursing supplementer
    150
removal from the breast 32–3
respiratory problems
  breastfeeding baby with
    119–20
  effect on feeding 16
  length of feed 35
retained placenta 93
rickets, neonatal 12
rooting 14, 117

scissor hold 82, *83*
silicon implant surgery 105
smoking 95, 163
sodium 12, 44
stools
  colour 132
  frequency 11
storage of expressed milk 56–7,
    71
sucking practice 36
sucking reflex 13, 14, 16
sucking, ineffective,
  cup-feeding and 147–8
supplementary and replacement
    (complementary) feeding
    69–71
  methods, types of 136
  necessity for 70–1
swallowing reflex 13, 14, 16
syringes 154–5, *154*

tension, effect on let-down reflex
    92
test weighing 103
thrush (*Candida albicans*) 76, 133
thyroid 93

tongue tie 15, 111, 128
trace elements in breastmilk 13
transpyloric tube, baby with 124,
    136–7
triglycerides 9
triplets
  milk supply 121
twins
  feeding position 31
  milk supply 121

unsettled baby
  reasons connected to
    breastfeeding 128
  reasons for 128
  solutions 129

vegans 12
ventilated baby 124–5
vitamin A 12
vitamin B complex 12
vitamin B6 12
vitamin C 12
vitamin D (calciferol) 12
  deficiency 12
  supplements 12
vitamin E 12, 79
vitamin K 12
vitamins in breastmilk 12

water in breastmilk 12
weight gain 38, 100, 102
weight loss 38, 103
  causes 103
  maternal 3
whey 11
woolwich shells 98

zinc 13